Ebola-iculous

Also by James Appel, MD

Nasara: Dispatches from a District Hospital in Chad

Children of the East: the Spiritual Heritage of Islam in the Bible

Messiah: the Jesus of the Qur'an and the Gospels

Ebola-iculous

A Physician Encounters the Ebola Capital of the World

James Appel, MD

You can obtain additional copies of this book by visiting
www.createspace.com/5031956

Bible verses marked NET are taken from the New English Translation Bible®
copyright ©1996-2006 by Biblical Studies Press, L.L.C. http://netbible.com
All rights reserved.

Front cover photo of pediatric patient at SDA Cooper Hospital
courtesy of James Appel

Back cover photo of SDA Cooper Hospital staff
courtesy of James Appel

Back author photo courtesy of James Appel

Photo of author and family courtesy of Heather Rice

Cover design by James Appel

Contact the author at appeltwin1@yahoo.com

Copyright © 2014 by James Appel, MD
All rights reserved.
ISBN-10: 1502700344
ISBN-13: 978-1502700346

FOR THE
COURAGEOUS
STAFF OF
THE SDA COOPER
HOSPITAL

As for you, the one who lives
in the shelter of the sovereign One...
he will certainly rescue you...
from the destructive plague...
You need not fear
the terrors of the night,...
the plague that comes in the darkness,
or the disease that comes at noon.
Though a thousand may fall beside you,
and a multitude on your right side,
it will not reach you...
No harm will overtake you;
no illness will come near your home.

PSALMS 91 (NET)

Contents

Ebola 05
Monrovia 09
Triage 15
Pee Pee 23
Symphysiotomy 27
Preshuh! 31
Sketchy 35
Bullet 39
Death 45
Pit 49
Sudden 53
Eyes 55
No Blood 59
Scars 63
Ebola-iculous 65
Interrogation 67
Deception 71
Stabbed 77
Body 81
Pregnancy 85
Blur 89
Liberianese 93
Conjunctiva 97
Shoulder 101
Stupid 105
Clues 107
Excision 113
Steve 117
Abortion 121
Fever 127
Paradise 131
Closed! 135
Limbo 139
Rain 143
Last Hurrah 145
Epilogue 149
Appendix 151
About the Author 155

Ebola
August 10-13

In all my medical training there's only been one thing that really scared me personally: Ebola. As you know, Ebola is running rampant across West Africa. Fortunately, it hasn't yet found it's way to the Republic of Chad where I've been living for the last 10 years.

However, sitting around in Yacoub's living room with a group of robed Muslim men, you'd have thought Ebola was lurking right around the corner. Everyone is panicked. They've heard that there are two cases in N'djamena. It has been announced that everyone should drink a half a glass of hot salt water before leaving home to protect themselves. Everyone wants to hear more. So I tell them what I know.

What I don't tell them is that the only reason I know anything is that since last night I've been doing serious research on it. Why? Because I'm going to be going into the heart of the epidemic in the Liberian capital of Monrovia.

Apparently, most of the hospitals in Monrovia have closed down because health care workers refuse to come to work and possibly expose themselves to Ebola. At first, it was even recommended that the surgeon at the Cooper Adventist Hospital be evacuated. However, Dr. Gillian refused to leave. As the only hospital in town doing surgery, she and her staff were being overrun with cases, especially by complicated obstetrics. How could she turn her back and just leave? She soon found herself working 18 hour days.

So, last night I was talking with my wife, Sarah, and she told me she'd just met with Dick Hart, Adventist Health International's president. Dick is wondering if I'm willing to go to Liberia to help for a few weeks to a month. My first reaction is abject fear. I've been following the story of the American doctor in Monrovia who almost died of Ebola. I'm well aware that Ebola has an up to 90% mortality rate, not to mention that there is no supposed treatment available except supportive care.

But I also don't believe in giving in to fear. I need to face this fear, especially since it is for such a good cause.

So Elisée and I pack up the ambulance and start the long drive across Chad on. That night I spend sleeping in the back of the ambulance parked outside the Catholic mission in Mongo. Elisée sleeps inside in the rented guest room. We continue on to N'Djamena the next day. The following day, I'm supposed board a flight to Ethiopia and then on to Monrovia. There are a few glitches in the plan. First, I have no Liberian visa. Second, I have a layover in Addis Ababa overnight and don't know where to stay. The Third one I'll only discover when I land in Accra.

The second is resolved when I get an email newsletter from my friends Adam and Michelle. They've just arrived in Addis Ababa to begin language study. They eventually will move south to work in a mission hospital.

They graciously agree to pick me up from the airport and let me spend the night. I exit the airport into the cold air of Addis and don't immediately see any cars at all, much less one with a friendly face.

I look out father and from way across some bushes and down a hill I see a tall American jumping up and down and yelling "James!" Boy, am I glad to see Adam!

I spend a pleasant evening eating grilled cheese sandwiches in Adam and Michelle's tiny apartment. I check my email next morning and finally get the invitation letter from Adventist Health International which I print out. At the time I don't realize how helpful this will turn out to be.

I have my boarding pass already for the flight to Ghana so I board the plane with no problem. I begin to panic on the flight. I know that Accra will be a challenge. For starters, I don't have a ticket. I also don't know if I'll need to get a Ghanian visa or not. Finally, I'm not sure they'll let me on the plane since I don't have a Liberian visa.

Gillian had emailed me last minute when I was still in N'Djamena and told me someone was working on getting someone to meet me at the airport, but nothing was confirmed. But even if I tell them that in Accra, why would they believe me? I have no proof.

Coming off the plane in Accra, I walk directly into the Customs line. There are no signs for transit passengers. Then I hear someone crying out "Transit! Transit!" I see a uniformed woman holding a list. I go up to her but my name is not on the transit list. I tell her I'm on the Kenyan Airlines for Monrovia.

The woman registers me by hand in a large book then gives me a laminated "tourist visa" card. Another uniformed woman then tells me to follow her.

There is an Indian man also going to Monrovia. We join up and follow our guide around Immigration and Customs. The Indian man picks up his bag at baggage claim. Then we walk outside and up a ramp to the entrance to the departure gates.

I go towards the Kenyan Airlines counter. At the front of the line, the man asks for my passport. He can't find my name on the list of passengers. My worst fears are coming true. I show him the email on my computer. He asks about my Liberian visa. I say I don't have one. He asks for some kind of paper. I pull out the Invitation Letter. He reads it, smiles, and says "Very good!" and waves me on.

At the counter, they can't find my name. Finally, they find out that my ticket has been voided. It's midnight in the USA so no way to call the travel agent. I offer to buy a new ticket. It comes to $484. No credit cards allowed. I have $400 with me. Then I remember I have some Euros in my wallet. I go to the exchange booth and get $90 for my 70 euros. Just enough to buy the ticket.

I finally am able to contact Dick Hart by telephone (fortunately, my Chadian SIM card works in Ghana). He says he'll call back after finding out what's going on from Gillian in Liberia. Finally, I get the call back confirming that they have a visa ready for me and will meet me at the airport!

Ebola, here I come!

Monrovia
August 14

I step out of the Kenya Airways jet and into the muggy air of Monrovia, the capital of Liberia. The sky is overcast with cracks of white letting in a little sunlight. The tarmac is wet from a recent rain. It's cool and breezy. Across the runway is a small airport with cracked paint on the walls. We get in a bus for the short trip to the door marked "Arrivals". A sign half falling off one of the double doors gives a list of the do's and don'ts for Ebola prevention.

We are let out of the bus in groups of ten. Right inside the door is a small man in a short white coat with a digital thermometer. He is taking the temperature of each arrival. As soon as each passenger is declared fever free they move to a water cooler constantly dripping chlorine impregnated water into a plastic bucket sitting on a stool.

Hand painted signs point us to one of three lines: "VIPs/Diplomates," "Liberians" or "Foreigners." I choose the appropriate line, passport without visa clutched nervously in my hand. I also hold a letter I just printed off that morning inviting me to come to Liberia as a relief physician for the Cooper Adventist Hospital, one of the few hospitals still open during the Ebola epidemic.

When it's my turn, I nervously go up to the Immigration booth and address the woman inside, talking through five holes haphazardly drilled through the plexiglass.

"I don't have a visa. Someone's supposed to meet me here to give me one."

Without saying a word she takes my passport and letter and walks out the back of the booth. Soon another woman comes up and says, "Follow me."

I go into a dingy back office with a desk piled with scattered papers. The woman shuffles through one pile and pulls out an official looking document with the words "Airport Visa" emblazoned in bold across the top. I'm relieved to see it has my name on it.

We go back to the booth where the first woman quickly stamps my passport and waves me through. I show my passport to the customs official who motions for me to go outside where a crowd has gathered. I see a few people with signs. None of them have my name. A man comes up to me and we start talking. I explain the situation, but he says he hasn't seen anyone from Cooper Hospital.

Just then a large man approaches from behind me and says in heavy Liberian English "Coopuh 'ospitawl???" He's holding a hand written sign that reads "SDA Cooper Hospital." I nod in relief and we weave our way through the sea of people waiting to leave Liberia. We approach a fairly new looking Land Cruiser hardtop with "Cooper Eye Hospital" written on the doors in green paint.

The driver introduces himself as Robert and soon has us rushing off on a nice paved road through lush tropical vegetation reminding me of a Latin America. Palms and banana trees poke out amidst the sprawling jungle interspersed with brightly colored wood or block houses and restaurants. But it's obvious for many miles that we are still in the country. In fact, it appears the airport is at least 30 miles from Monrovia.

As we approach the city, we pass a huge walled compound to the left, just between the road and the ocean. "Dat's de ELWA 'ospitawl," says my host, who has identified himself as an immigration officer but who is an Adventist Church member.

The ELWA Hospital is where the Ebola cases are being referred to and where the American Doctor and Nurse stricken with the disease were cared for. For over a week the staff kept them alive with IV fluids and electrolyte replacement. They finally also were given an experimental mix of monoclonal antibodies called ZMapp. Whether Zmapp was the deciding factor or not is debatable, but they recovered enough to be evacuated to the United States where they are making a recovery.

ELWA is also where one of my former attending physicians from residency, John Fankhauser, is spearheading the medical care of the Ebola patients in their treatment center.

Robert continues his mad pace as we enter the capital. Monrovia is like so many cities in the developing world: crowded, a mix of modern and primitive. lots of cars, but no electricity unless you have your own personal generator.

We stay on the main road for a long time through town until we turn right on some pothole filled road. After a couple blocks, Robert stops the Land Cruiser in front of a dilapidated building with "SDA Cooper Hospital" emblazoned over the front doors leading from a small circular parking space. All the staff is sitting outside on a low wall.

I soon find out why. Two days previously, the rumor had got out that the Cooper Hospital also had an Ebola case, so patients had stopped coming. Today, though, a real suspicious case had come through and just died in the hallway. The patient had been sick for a week with fever and vomiting. He went to ELWA hospital who saw that he also had an incarcerated hernia. Instead of first checking him for Ebola, they sent him straight over to Cooper.

Dr. Gillian Seton, the hospital's surgeon, was doing triage on patients at the time. She was suspicious but also felt he should be examined for his hernia. She took precautions and allowed no one else around the patient, gloved up and was able to reduce the hernia. Then the patient vomited on her arm and died.

The body was quickly doused in chlorine and wrapped in plastic bags and OR wraps. The staff then moved the cadaver to the unused X-ray room and plopped it on a bench. Everything was then properly dosed with chlorine water and clothes disposed of. The Ministry of Health was called to evacuate the body and test it for Ebola. No one has come yet.

The staff are refusing to go back in the hospital. The doors are temporarily shut to new patients. Robert introduces me to some of the staff and then I meet Gillian. Her extended hand marks the last time anyone will shake my hand for weeks. People are afraid of any physical contact.

Gillian takes me and shows me my room. It's inside the compound on a courtyard under the operating theater and Labor and Delivery room upstairs. The compound feels crowded with a lot of buildings crammed in a small space.

The rooms were the dwelling of a Filipino couple who've just left on annual leave. She was the staff OB/GYN and he worked in accounting. The cabinets are sagging, half the drawers are swollen shut by the humidity, small cockroaches abound, and most of the furniture is about to fall over. The couch and chairs are nice though, as is the bed and mattress.

Gillian brings me some excellent pasta and a Greek salad from a nearby restaurant. I'm starved so I make short work of the late supper. I haven't really eaten well in the four days since I left Abeche in Eastern Chad to cross the desert, head to Eastern Africa and then fly almost the length of the upper horn of Africa to Liberia.

I feel much better with a full belly and despite the pit in my stomach caused by my fear of Ebola and the unknown, I fall into a deep sleep.

The next morning, I awaken and prepare breakfast. I quickly down yoghurt, oatmeal and a peanut butter and jelly sandwich. I walk out to the lobby where I meet and talk with many of the staff.

The dead body from yesterday is still in the X-ray room. The Ministry of Health has shown no signs of action despite being called continually by our administration. I'm told that in at least one case, they took 5 days before they came for a body in one neighborhood. By leaving the cadaver, many more people were exposed. One of the main ways Ebola is transmitted is through contact with dead bodies.

Staff worship is upstairs on the wards at 8:00AM. After worship, I accompany Gillian on rounds. In the middle of rounds, we are told the family has come to reclaim the body. Our medical director, Dr. Sonii has a devious plan: let the family take the body, but inform the police who will wait for them around the corner. The police will to arrest the family, take the body to test it and then bury it safely in a secret grave site reserved for Ebola victims.

The family is dressed in a typical Muslim fashion. They pull a beat up small pickup into the side yard near the outdoor kitchen. Some soup is being boiled over a wood fire on a grill.

The three pallbearers are called up to the hallway just outside the X-ray room. Gillian explains how to put on the protective gear given us by the Ministry of Health. The men zip on full body suits. They pull booties over the bottoms of the suits. When they put on the two pairs of gloves we realize the sleeves are too short. The sleeves pull out easily from under the gloves leaving the wrists exposed!

Gillian solves the problem with her pocket knife. She cuts thumb holes in the sleeves which are looped over the thumbs before reapplying the gloves. Now the sleeves stay under the gloves. We give the men heavy duty masks as the final piece of their protective armor. Gillian then instructs them how to remove the gear when they're done, placing it safely in the red biohazard bags. This is an obvious weakness in the system and the likelihood of contamination is high.

The three men go into the X-ray room and pick up the whole bench where the corpse has been laid. They take body and bench through the hallway, down a flight of stairs, past the kitchen and into the open air where the truck waits.

Meanwhile, I've spread a large impermeable OR drape in the bed of the truck to hopefully contain the bodily fluids which may or may not be filled with the Ebola virus. The pallbearers lift the whole bench into the truck bed and then slip the body onto the drape, remove the bench and wrap the body up in the rest of the sheet.

I look at the bench placed to the side. There is a huge wet spot under where the man's abdomen and thorax had been. His bodily fluids have soaked into the wood. The truck drives outside and Gillian goes upstairs to prepare the death certificate. I spray some chlorine water on the bench's wettest spots and then go upstairs.

There seems to be a new problem now. The head of the family states that they can't go out dressed as biohazard personnel. They'll be arrested immediately (of course, that's the point, but we can't say that).

So now we have to have them come back in the courtyard, take off their suits and give them new suits to put on once they get to the graveyard. I doubt they'll use them. As the men remove their suits there is a lot of cross contamination and general chaos.

They wash their hands in diluted bleach water, hop in the back of the pickup and take off. I use the rest of the bucket of chlorine water to douse the entire bench. When I'm done with the top, I grab a stick from the ground to push the bench over so I can soak the bottom as well.

I wash up well and Gillian and I finish rounds. There aren't many patients because of the earlier scare. There are no admissions or surgeries the rest of the day.

I spend the afternoon talking to Gillian about the challenges of the Cooper Hospital and after a hefty supper of lentils, rice and fried plantains I go to my room. I wash my clothes by hand, hang them up in the bathroom and living room, take a shower and fall into a deep sleep.

Triage
August 16

    Here in Liberia things don't start as early as in Chad, at least not at the Cooper Hospital. After a quick breakfast of yogurt and a peanut butter and jelly sandwich, I head out the front door into the small courtyard with the three story hospital just to the left. I squeeze through a narrow passageway between the wall and a flight of steps up to another Gillian's apartment. I turn right into a dim corridor with the open air kitchen just ahead opening to the other side of the building. I turn left half way down and go up two half-flights of stairs to the main hallway.

    Patients are already lining up outside, but I continue upstairs two more half flights to the wards. I come in just in time for staff worship. When it's done Gillian and I go downstairs and she shows me the triage area.

    Because of the Ebola outbreak, we screen for any suspected cases before they enter our hospital. Our primary objective is to keep our doors open so we can take care of the non-Ebola emergencies. The ELWA hospital on the other side of town is taking care of the Ebola patients. If I let in one case I not only put myself at risk, but the patients and staff as well. And if we get one staff member sick with Ebola we'll close down like all the other hospitals. No one will have anywhere to go when they're sick.

    So, we don't let patients inside without being screened. We set up a small table with two chairs on the front porch. When patients come, we find out where they are from and their names. If they come from a village with a major outbreak that should be quarantined, they are turned away automatically.

    Then we ask the potential patients about symptoms that could suggest Ebola: fever, headache, sore throat, vomiting, diarrhea, coughing or any kind of bleeding. If they don't look sick and have less then 3 of the above symptoms, we send them in to be registered. Afterwards, they come back outside. Then they are called in for vital signs and the chart put in the consultant's office. Finally, we call them in and consult them. The diagnosis is made almost exclusively on history as a physical exam involving touching a patient puts everyone at risk for this pestilence transmitted by contact. At last, we prescribe medications for the patients and they go home.

Shortly after I start putting this triage into practice, a cab pulls up. There's a woman inside, very pregnant and obviously not doing well. A man jumps out of the car carrying a note from a health center. It says she's been in labor for two days and is bleeding, hypotensive and has no fetal presenting part. I go to the cab, putting on gloves as I go. I reach in the back door and palpate her abdomen. I feel fetal parts and instantly suspect a ruptured uterus. After asking her the standard Ebola screening questions, I find her to be low risk. I call for a wheelchair to take her up to surgery.

I'm still not registered with the Liberian Medical and Dental Council so I can't operate yet. Gillian takes over and calls in the OR team. I go back down to triage. I have just started the screening process when Mrs. Carter, the administrator and Dr. Sonii, the medical director come up.

They say it might be trouble if I'm seen working without permission from the council. They suggest I get my papers together and they'll take it over immediately and see if they can steamroll the process. I find some copies of the necessary documents on my computer, others I've brought from Chad, while still others I have to compose and print out. I also give them two of the passport photos I'd taken yesterday in the market.

Dr. Sonii takes the whole packet over to the Ministry of Health and soon comes back saying they've ok'd me to start working even though they won't get all the paperwork finished until next week.

So I find myself back doing triage. Soon another taxi pulls up. A man hurries up with a flaccid preteen in his arms. I now have a nurse's aide and an intern, Dr. Scotland, helping me. R.B., the nurse's aide, makes them take him back quickly and put him in the back seat of the cab. I put on gloves and go over to take a look.

The family claims the boy was just hanging up laundry on the line and got electrocuted. Apparently, the close line was really a power line.

R.B. steps back and says "He not breathin', doctuh."

I verify that there is no pulse or respiratory effort and pronounce him dead. His mother starts flopping around screaming and holding her head. I take off my gloves and go back to triage.

I finish with the outpatients by noon and go to see what's happening with the c-section. Gillian has just finished and is writing her operative note. The anesthetist and OR assistant are transferring the patient to the gurney. She is still unconscious and floppy. They move her immediately to the wards. There is no post-op recovery room at the hospital.

After she's in her bed I examine her conjunctiva and find them extremely pale, almost white. She has lost a lot of blood. There is no blood bank but they've been working on getting family members to donate. The relatives are refusing. Someone has gone across town and bought a bag of blood from somewhere. We get that running as fast as possible but She has only one IV, a small one in her left hand.

Alex, the nurse, rechecks her blood pressure. She is still hypotensive and has a fast pulse. The midwife, Dede, and Alex are both trying to find an IV, even attempting the veins on her feet and ankles. There is no access. The blood is running in very slowly and finally stops altogether. The tubing is clotted off.

Alex runs to the pharmacy and returns with another set of transfusion tubing. The hospital has no central line kits so we are trying to get a regular IV in the femoral vein. I finally get the catheter into the vein but it's very position dependent. I have to sit there holding the catheter while IV fluids pour in.

Another bag of blood finally comes. The woman is still unconscious. Finally, her pulse slows down some, but is still too rapid. The blood pressure has improved as well. Gillian has Alex call the family to try and get more blood. At least we have two good IV's running now with a unit of blood running in each one.

I take a break and go eat a late lunch of spaghetti and cucumber salad. It's late afternoon by now. After lunch, I go relax a little, take a shower and do some laundry by hand. Leter, I Skype with Sarah and the kids, the first time I've seen them in about a month. Then I go to bed.

I toss and turn all night. I'm worried about the woman with the uterine rupture and Ebola keeps lurking in my nightmares as a constant veiled threat. Finally, I fall asleep at about 3:00AM and wake up after 7:30AM. A half hour later, Gillian comes to the door.

"The woman coded last night. Fortunately, the nurse called me in time and we were able to give her adrenaline and more blood. She pulled through. I've been up all night, though, and am exhausted. There's two c-sections to be done, can you do them?"

"Sure, that's why I'm here..."

I've started making French toast but only have one prepared. I down that one quickly and go up to Labor and Delivery following the same maze of dim passageways that at first was confusing but is already becoming familiar.

Dede is still on duty. She's been on for almost 48 hours since no one came to relieve her yesterday evening. Many of the staff refuse to come in, scared of getting Ebola. Dede seems to know her stuff and is very conscientious from what I've seen. I'm glad to see her.

"What's going on?" I ask.

"Dis woman, she been he-uh since yestuhday. She not progressin' in huh laybuh and now de fetal heaht rate not raht. I put huh on huh left side an' de heaht rate improvin'."

"This is the woman with a hemoglobin of 8 from yesterday right?"

"Yeah, doc."

Gillian has called in the OR team already and they're on their way. I go to the lab to make sure we have blood. They have one bag already, but it looks like it's in a pediatric blood bag which is only half the volume of an adult bag. The hospital is out of adult sizes.

I come back upstairs and the OR team is assembled in the changing room putting on scrubs. I reach out my hand and shake the hand of a large man with a toothy grin who introduces himself as Mr. Wezzeh (pronounced "Wheezy".) A large, stocky man with a weathered face then speaks up.

"Hey man, dis Ebola time. We don' shake hands. Go wash."

I laugh and comply. The man then introduces himself as News (pronounced like Neal with a nasal ending), the anesthetist. Joseph, the circulating nurse and instrument specialist nods from the corner as he pulls on his scrub top. I pull on the surgical cap I brought from Chad, put on a mask and head into the operating theater. It's small, but clean and seems well equipped, although there's only one ancient OR light and most of the equipment looks like it may have survived the Second World War.

"What anesthesia will you use?" I ask News.

"General."

"What about spinal?"

To me it's a simple question but it brings forth an aggressive response from News as if I'd insulted his mother. He goes on and on about how he knows what he's doing and a spinal would not be right in this case since the patient has anemia and he's worked in Britain and who am I to question him, etc, etc, etc.

I'm a bit taken aback by his reply, but bite my tongue. I'm already wary of his abilities based on his poor handling of the uterine rupture from yesterday but I don't say anything. I go downstairs and find some long shoe covers to protect my feet and legs from exposure to bodily fluids and head back up. News is just coming out of Labor and Delivery and confronts me again aggressively.

"You happy wit' my anesthesia or not? Huh? Jus' le' me know, ok?"

I motion him over away from the rest of the staff into the changing room where we are alone.

"Listen, News, I'm not sure why you are being so defensive. I was just asking a question. For me, that's good medical practice. One should dialogue, communicate and discuss and that's all I was trying to do."

"Ok, man, ok. You say you always done c-sections under spinal and you like dem because dey relax the lower abdomen. So will my general. You never try a c-section under general, le' me show you how it work."

Deep down, I'm not satisfied, but it's not the time to pick a fight. I nod and we move into the theater again. The patient is already on the table. I notice she just has a small 20G IV in her left hand and an even tinier 22G in her right antecubital fossa.

I mention to News that I'd like at least one 18G IV line before doing surgery. He doesn't say anything as he hangs up the bag of blood and gets it ready to give. I don't push but watch him warily out of the corner of my eye. He doesn't start another IV and then I notice the 22G isn't even working at all. I reluctantly don't say anything.

"Go scrub!" orders News.

I comply. At first, all I see are hard, plastic scrub brushes used normally for cleaning instruments. There are also some old bars of soap on the counter. I then see a blue covered dish. I open the lid carefully and inside see two used regular surgical scrub brushes. One seems to still have some chlorhexadine on it so I scrub with that.

After my scrub, I back through the swinging doors of the theater, my hands held out in front of my chest high and well away from my body. I pick up a small washcloth folded lying on the surgical gown and wipe my hands dry. I then fully dry them in front of the A/C and put on my gown and gloves in sterile fashion.

The woman's exposed, very pregnant belly is covered in some kind of substance that looks like fine wood chips. I've seen this many times in Chad. It's some kind of traditional medicine. I have the circulating nurse wash it off with soap and water before prepping with Betadine.

"Doctuh James," News begins, apparently ready with some more advice for me. "De fastuh you do dis section de better for you and for me…"

"...and for the patient and the infant." I add dryly.

"Yeah, o' course," News quickly agrees.
"I always consider c-sections under these conditions to be crash c-sections...So I always do them as fast as possible." I add.
"Yeah, an' now I'll show you crash anesthesia too," adds News with an evil gleam in his eye.
We've draped the patient's abdomen and I stand poised with the scalpel after surveying the instrument tray and finding most of what I'd expect in a c-section kit (although I'd really prefer more than 2 ring clamps).
"News, can I start?"
"O' course, jus' waitin' for you."
"Le's pray fuhst," interjects Mr. Wezzeh who'll be assisting me. "Dee-uh Gawd i' de name o' Jeeesus, we tank you fo' de muh-cees, fo' dis opuhrashun, fo'de healin's i' de name o' Jeeesus....Ahhh-men!"
"Amen!" I echo and slice down quickly through skin, fat, fascia and peritoneum. The woman moans and contracts her muscles. She's still feeling it! So much for "crash anesthesia!"
"She's moving!" I tell News.
I pull open the wound with my hands, extend it inferiorly with scissors. I have to fight against the intestines wanting to push their way out thanks to the tight abdominal muscles that would've been relaxed with a spinal anesthetic. I force in the bladder blade but have a hard time seeing the lower uterine segment as Mr. Wezzeh and I continue our struggle against the powers of this present operation.
Finally, I am able to get a bladder flap developed and retract the bladder out of the way. I make a small incision in the uterus, poke through with a clamp and extend it to both sides and superiorly with my fingers and scissors. The baby's head is right there.
"Push on the top of the uterus!" I tell Mr. Wezzeh. His efforts are less than adequate so I reach my left hand up and push down hard as my right hand guides the head out. A flexing baby with excellent muscle tone who seems to want to cry emerges. I quickly wipe him off while Mr. Wezzeh clamps and cuts the cord.
I hand the baby off to Dede. I turn back to the deliver the placenta. In the back of my mind, I'm still listening in vain for that reassuring newborn cry. I tug too hard on the umbilical cord and it pops off the placenta. No big deal. I reach my hand in the uterus and scrape the placenta off the uterine wall then exteriorize the uterus.

There is a bleeding artery on the left that I clamp with one of the two ring clamps and then grasp the other edges of the uterine incision with some other clamps.

I still don't hear the baby cry.

I look over and Dede is bringing a limp newborn over to News who is getting a bag valve mask ready.

"Start chest compressions!" I order.

"De chil' ha' a hahtbeat, he jus' not breathin," replies News in his husky voice that's growing more irritating by the minute.

"How fast is the heartbeat, if it's under a hundred beats per minute that's not good enough. And chest compressions will move air into the lungs in the meantime as well. It certainly won't hurt."

News smiles condescendingly and continues doing what he's doing. I turn back to the mother. She's my first priority. Hopefully, the baby will make it despite the lack of protocol. I suture the uterus and after assuring that the bleeding is controlled replace it into the abdomen.

I verify that there is no bleeding from the wound and close the fascia. I finally hear a weak baby cry. Thank God! I close the skin with a flimsy, tapered needle more suited to thin bowel than tough skin. Eventually I'm able to finish the job with a very warped needle at the end.

I scrub out and thank News who thanks me back. As I leave the room, I hear News bragging to Mr. Wezzeh: "See, I tol' you dat general anesthesia de bes'…"

I pretend not to hear as I walk out and almost bump into Gillian.

"The woman with the ruptured uterus from yesterday just died."

Life and death.

Pee Pee

August 18

"He not pee pee free fo' twoo week." The father seems to beg me with his eyes to do something as he answers my question as to why he and his wife have brought their newborn son to the Cooper Hospital.

I'm sitting outside in the screening area to try and identify patients with Ebola symptoms so we can refer them to the ELWA Hospital where they can be isolated and tested. We can't afford for our patients and staff to be exposed to Ebola. This child obviously has a different problem.

I take the small family to my office and have the mother take off the layers of homemade diaper she's fabricated out of a plastic bag covering some rags.

A boy's traumatized penis emerges from the wrappings. What's left of the foreskin is jagged, swollen and bloody with the glans barely peeking through some ratty ends of purple suture. His abdomen is tense and distended with prominent, dilated veins above the belly button.

"When was he circumcised?" I ask the father.

"It been twoo week," he replies.

"Since the circumcision he hasn't gone pee pee?"

"No."

"Was he able to pee pee before the circumcision?"

"Yeah, small, small."

"He can poo poo? He breastfeeds normally?"

"Yeah, he tryin'."

"What's his name?"

"Moses," shyly replies the mother.

I find a suture kit and with the scissors and forceps remove the sutures from the tiny penis. The site of the stitching starts to ooze. The suture was obviously compressing the tip of the penis.

Now that I've freed it up I expect something to happen, but Moses still doesn't pee. I gently press on the distended bladder. Nothing. I go to search for a small urinary catheter. The smallest I can find is a 10F. It's way too big.

Gillian and I go search in the chaotic stockroom. We find a single use red robbin catheter that is 8F. I try to insert it but it's too big as well.

Suddenly, Gillian remembers some suction catheters for ET tubes. We find one that's 6F. I cut off the paraphernalia surrounding the tube and with a lot of lubrication get it to go in part way into the boy's tiny urethra. I twist and turn and gently probe until finally it bursts into the bladder and over 300cc of dark brown urine comes out. The abdomen becomes a normal pudgy newborn belly. Moses and his parents are obviously relieved.

"Tank you Lawd, tank you Lawd! Tank you Jeeesus!" exclaims the father, a huge smile on his face. The mother sits quietly with a silly grin on her face.

Now I'm faced with the fact that this tube has no balloon to make sure it doesn't come out. I decide to see if Moses can now pee on his own with the release of the suture constricting the urethra. I take the tube out, give him a shot of Ceftriaxone (which I administer myself since we have no nursing staff), and tell them to come back tomorrow.

The next morning, I see the mother sitting out in the crowded waiting room. It seems patients have decided to come back today. The waiting room is packed. I have the Paul, one of the physician's Assistants screen them for signs of Ebola.

I walk up to the baby's mother. "Has Moses gone pee pee?" I ask.

The mother shakes her head "No" as she removes the diaper, this time a real diaper. Moses' abdomen is swollen again, but the edema of the abdominal wall is gone. The kidneys are functioning well despite the obstruction!

I reinsert another suction tube, drain over 300 more milliliters of clearer urine and this time leave the tube in. The penis is much less swollen and starting to look almost normal. I still give one more shot of Ceftriaxone and tell them to come back tomorrow. I hope that if the tube can stay in at least 24 hours then the bladder can stay shrunken down and Moses will start to feel the need to pee before it gets too distended.

In the meantime, Paul calls me to evaluate two patients who've come by taxi. The first one is an elderly woman sitting motionless in the back seat, her face covered by a head scarf. Her legs are exposed revealing old sores on her ankles and feet with some edema.

The family says she hasn't pooped in 5 days. Her belly is somewhat swollen but not tense. I remove the head scarf and she looks like death warmed over. My radar is on high alert. I can't take the risk that she might have Ebola. I tell the family there's nothing we can do.

The relatives protest. They show me a torn slip of paper with the name "Dr. Gunnar" and phone number on it with a note in chicken scratch saying "not suspicious for Ebola." That makes me more suspicious and I insist they leave.

It's hard to do, my whole medical training screams "No!" But I know I have to protect the staff and patients in order to keep the hospital open. If we admit even one Ebola patient, none of the staff or patients will come and many others will die who could be helped.

The next cab has a middle aged man in it. He is awake but doesn't talk or look at me. The son tells me he had been having black, tarry stools but now is constipated for the last 6 days. I look at his conjunctiva with a gloved finger and the under eyelids are very red.

I also feel uneasy. It's a gut feeling. Bleeding is a prominent feature of Ebola. They may be lying about diarrhea, vomiting and fever. I offer to give them some ulcer medicine (in case that's the cause of his bloody stools) and some laxatives (in case it's only constipation). They really want to be admitted. They say he won't eat and won't take pills. I say I'm sorry and send them away with some tablets.

I screen some more unsuspicious patients and then they bring in a six year old girl who is obviously sick. No diarrhea, but she has fever, abdominal pain and vomiting. I'm suspicious but also realize it could be just malaria.

She throws up some thick, bilious vomit in a small amount into the bed pan. I'm wearing gloves of course. I instantly rinse out the bed pan and soak everything in chlorine water.

I prescribe Artemether injections twice a day for her possible malaria and Ceftrixone injections for her possible typhoid. Inside my head, I pray that she does't have Ebola and that the injections will work. As soon as she leaves I wipe everything down with a chlorine soaked rag and have the cleaning team come in and decontaminate the floor.

I go eat a quick lunch while they are decontaminating the room. I come back just in time to see the Paul putting in a ten year old boy who is wearing only a ragged pair of shorts soaked in urine or some other bodily fluid. I quickly learn that he was brought in urgently by his mom who carried him in on his back because he's too weak to walk. He's had fever and vomiting for several days.

"GET HIM OUT OF HERE!" I yell. "THESE ARE EXACTLY THE KINDS OF CASES THAT WE ARE SCREENING FOR!"

Just then the mother let's out a wail. The child is dead. She grabs the boy and runs out. I continue to explain in a loud voice to all the staff that patients with these kinds of symptoms are the ones that are supposed to be screened and sent away.

"But he too sick to be screened outsahde," replies Paul, weakly trying to defend his actions. "Paul, it's exactly the sickest ones that are the most dangerous to us and to our other patients. And in the end, we didn't help him at all. He died! We just put ourselves at risk!"

We close the room. Aaron from housekeeping dons complete gowns, gloves, masks, boots, and masks. Then he pulverizes and sterilizes the room. We leave it off limits the rest of the day.

The struggle against Ebola continues.

Symphysiotomy
August 19

The baby is back, little baby Moses who can't pee pee. Of course, the catheter I put in yesterday has come out. The mother brings it with her. I sterilize it in diluted bleach water and reinsert it into the tiny bladder. Now that the staff is all back to work, I admit the baby so we can keep an eye on the catheter and put it back in quickly if it comes out. We want that distended bladder to shrink back down to normal so Moses will feel the urge to pee pee before his bladder gets ridiculously huge.

Yesterday, we had a staff meeting with almost all of the 90 or so staff present. It seems there was confusion about a lot of things. But in the end, the leaders were inspiring and everyone's questions were answered, so most have returned to work. It's such a different feel with a full staff. I don't feel so alone and running around like a chicken with its head cut off.

Gillian and I continue to share the load of screening patients outside. I happen to be outside when a yellow taxi pulls up and about 5 people pile out, including an obviously pregnant woman howling in pain. I ask her the typical screening questions which are all negative. Despite her screams of pain, she's obviously in good overall health. I quickly admit her to labor and delivery. It's her second pregnancy. The first was delivered by c-section for having cephalopelvic disproportion (pelvis too small, baby's head to big.) This will be a perfect case for a pubic symphysiotomy.

The midwives get her set up on the delivery table, start an IV and try to get in a urinary catheter. Gillian gets the instruments, suture, scalpel blade and lidocaine. I am able to insert the foley catheter by pushing up on the fetal head between contractions. The head is very deformed and the cervix is dilated completely. Ideal indications and conditions for the symphysiotomy.

I clean the front of the pelvis and groin with chlorhexadine and inject down to the cartilage that holds the pelvic bones together in front. I slip my fingers inside to displace the foley catheter (and thus the urethra) to one side and also to give me a sense of depth perception so I don't cut too deep. With my right hand I make a skin incision and then cut down directly to the cartilage. Slowly and methodically I slice through the cartilage layer by layer. It's all by feel and I stop periodically to feel where I am with my index finger. Finally, I have my two assistants pull the hips up and out and the pelvic bones separate 2-3cm.

"Stop!" I order once I feel the appropriate separation.

I fold open a piece of gauze and stuff it into the bleeding wound for hemostasis. The baby's head has already descended and with three good pushes the baby comes out looking like a cone head with bulging eyes from being compressed in the narrow birth canal.

I use the bulb suction to aspirate the gunk from the baby's mouth and nose. It's a boy! I place him on his mommy's belly where I clean and dry him before cutting the umbilical cord. His eyes are open and he's breathing but kind of floppy and not as pink as I'd like. His cry is weak. We stimulate, dry, suck and finally take him to the OR for oxygen before I'm happy with his skin color, muscle tone and cry.

I gently pull out the placenta and Gillian sutures up the wound. The mother keeps smiling and thanking God.

I go back to the Outpatient Department and see a few patients. One of the Physician's Assistants calls me in to see someone. He's had severe right lower quadrant pain since yesterday morning. He hasn't been vomiting but otherwise his history and physical seem to confirm the PA's suspicion of acute appendicitis. The weird thing is he came in yesterday afternoon and the PA told him to come back today since we were all in a meeting. I would've been fine seeing him yesterday evening. Oh well. I ask Gillian to confirm and she agrees and takes him to the operating theater.

I go back to screening patients. Just as we are about to close for the evening, another cab pulls up. Inside is an unconscious man with labored breathing. He has a history of hypertension and yesterday received a call that his son had died in another town. He kind of went crazy and started to go downhill culminating in a coma since this morning. He doesn't look otherwise sick and the family denies fever, vomiting and diarrhea so I admit him.

Our lab can't even check a blood sugar but I think the man might be hypoglycemic. I start an infusion of IV Dextrose. His blood pressure is surprisingly not that high. His malaria smear is negative. Then he starts seizing. I suspect he's having a hemorrhagic stroke and I know there's really nothing to do. But I give him some diazepam to stop the seizure, put him on IV fluids and leave him in the hospital bed, sending a quick prayer his way as I leave.

I go downstairs just in time to meet a group of women running up to the hospital. The lead woman holds a floppy infant in her arms. I quickly examine the conjunctiva with a gloved finger. They are pale white. He's anemic. After quickly determining he hasn't had vomiting or diarrhea I ask more questions about his history. Last week his mom took him to a health center. They told her he had anemia and malaria and gave him some pills.

I admit him for a blood transfusion and appropriate malaria treatment. The ER nurse quickly finds an IV, the lab is on the case and quickly testing some of the women for potential donors. I order an Artemether shot while the Quinine drip is being set up. The case is pretty hopeless but I've seen many similar patients pull through in Chad.

I go home, emotionally and physically exhausted. Having the spectra of Ebola hanging over us is a weighty affair. Just yesterday, a group of thieves looted an Ebola isolation unit, stealing mattresses and linens and causing 26 suspected Ebola cases to flee into the city.

People have written me emails saying nothing should really be done because compared to the big killers—malaria, TB and HIV—Ebola is barely killing anyone. What people aren't seeing from the comfort of their faraway living room chairs is that schools, businesses, government offices and hospitals are closed.

Money is getting scarce. Our hospital hasn't been paid in months by the insurance companies and is running low on generator fuel and supplies. People are dying more often than usual of treatable diseases because many hospitals are closed. Plus, they are afraid to come in to any hospitals that are open for fear of catching Ebola. Therefore, they are waiting too long at home. When things get serious, the family drives around getting refused by most clinics and hospitals until the patient if at death's door by the time they arrive at Cooper Hospital, if they make it here at all.

The country is about to fail financially because of the epidemic. As if they didn't already have enough problems. But some claim we shouldn't do anything about Ebola anyway because only about 1000 people or so have died. The number of deaths is only the tip of the ice burg when talking about the devastating effects of Ebola.

I fall into a restless sleep filled with nightmares.

Preshuh!

August 20

I go outside the hospital to see the man in the taxi. He's young and looks like very recently he was strong and healthy.

"What's his age?" I ask.

"Twenty year."

Now, he's looking like death warmed over. First glance show's he's in a coma, with foamy saliva coming out his mouth and swollen protruding eyes.

"How long has he been sick?"

"Since yestuhday he got preshuh, his hea' can huht him, he say he got pain in his hea'."

After confirming he has no vomiting, fever, cough, diarrhea, bleeding or other signs of Ebola, I call for a blood pressure cuff. I'm skeptical that a twenty year old really has "preshuh". I need to confirm or I'll send him away. Amazingly, his blood pressure is astronomically high: 248/148!

I have the family bring him in the hospital. I suspect he may have thyroid storm, where his thyroid hormone is raging out of control. Our lab cannot confirm. We can't do thyroid function tests.. We have no IV medicine, but he is awake enough to swallow some pills to lower his blood pressure and slow his fast heart rate. I also administer some iodine drops to help slow down his thyroid (if that's the problem.) He goes upstairs with further orders for IV fluids and steroids.

Another woman is out in the parking lot in a private vehicle. She also has "preshuh." She is in a coma, foaming at the mouth and breathing shallow. According to her family, she has no other symptoms. She heard that her daughter had died in another village, became agitated and then slowly slipped into a coma. Her blood pressure is "only" 160/92 but I suspect a stroke, probably hemorrhagic, with cerebral edema.

There's not much hope for her, but the family is desperate for something to be done. They've been turned away at several other health facilities already. I have the nurses start two IV's and get her upstairs. Before I can even go up and check on her, the nurses come down to tell me she has "passed." I go up and confirm her death, fill out the death certificate and the family soon brings in a van to take the body away.

I go to round on some of the patients from yesterday. The boy with severe anemia and malaria who was brought in almost dead is awake, alert and eating. Gillian tells me the little baby Moses' urinary catheter has come out again and he still can't pee pee. I have the pharmacy manager, Mrs. Wennie, try and locate a small foley catheter with a balloon that will stay in. I promise to come back later to put in the urinary catheter.

I go back to screening incoming patients for Ebola. There are no suspicious cases. A man comes in a yellow cab. He is elderly, frail and weak, yet alert. He has some edema in his lower legs and the family says he has "heart problems." He's followed normally every month at another hospital that is currently closed. Yesterday, he started feeling weak. He has no other symptoms.

I listen to his heart. It has a regular rhythm with some skipped beats and an impressive murmur suggesting a problem with his aortic valve, probably stenosis. I bring him in and check his blood pressure. The pulse pressure is wide at 120/40 in both arms. I'm not sure I can do much, but I order some IV fluids, a malaria smear, a typhoid test, a hemoglobin and have the family bring me his home medications. He goes upstairs to the wards. The results of the tests come back normal.

I go upstairs to check on the young man I admitted with severe hypertensive emergency. He looks like death warmed over. He became agitated and is now restrained with cords around his ankles and wrists tied to the bed. He also got Diazepam. Now he has swallow breathing and is foaming at the mouth. His eyes are still bulging and edematous. I Alex to put in a foley catheter and give him some Lasix.

Then as I'm palpating his pulse, it disappears. I call down the hallway for help and Gillian and a couple nurses come running. Someone brings the "crash cart" which is a carton of supplies Gillian has put together for emergencies. We do CPR, give him adrenaline several times, bag him, and get a heart beat back for a few minutes with some spontaneous respirations.

Then the breathing goes again. I intubate him and continue CPR but bloody froth is pouring out his nose and the ET tube. Finally, soaked in sweat, I stop and pronounce him dead. His uncle has observed the whole thing. Gillian asks if he has any questions. He replies that he saw the whole thing and seems satisfied that we've done our best. We pull out all the tubes and IV's and cover up his face.

I go back to pediatrics and am able to reinsert the urinary catheter and drain Baby Moses' bladder. The urine is now clear and pale yellow only. The inflammation from the circumcision is all but gone and he has no more edema. It seems Moses' kidneys have fully recovered. Mrs. Wennie has searched all around town for hours with no luck in finding a real foley catheter.

I go into the OR where Gillian is doing her second D&C of the day. She's finished the procedure but the patient is in respiratory distress. Her blood pressure was slightly high on entering the OR. She is one week out from delivery, maybe she had pre-eclampsia. After the case, it skyrocketed to 220/130 and she started breathing fast. She then told Gillian she has asthma.

As I walk in, she is getting a breathing treatment and has already gotten several doses of Lasix for pulmonary edema. he is sitting on the OR table, morbidly obese, with nasal flaring, sub costal retractions and labored breathing. Her eyes are open but staring a little wildly as she inhales the nebulizer treatment in shallow breaths. She also has severe pitting edema of her lower extremities. I listen to her lungs and she has tight wheezes, crackles and barely any air movement.

"Let's give her 80mg of Lasix this time and put in a foley catheter." I order Joseph who quickly gets working.

I'm nervous about a repeat of the young man from earlier. This time, though, the Lasix works. When Joseph gets the foley in, 1500ml comes out immediately. Joseph empties the bag and I give her more albuterol nebulizer treatments. The urine bag quickly fills with another 1500ml. She is breathing easier.

"I wanna eat! I wanna drink!" The woman is insistent, speaking in gasping breaths. Maybe she's hypoglycemic? Mr. Wezzeh brings her some juice which she gulps down eagerly. He also gives her some water and a sugar cube.

Meanwhile her lungs start to clear up even though her blood pressure stays high. Finally, 5 minutes after drinking the juice and eating the sugar cube her pressure starts to come down. Meanwhile, another 1300ml has come out in the urine bag! Her leg edema is starting to go down to. I'm afraid now she'll get low potassium from all the diuresis.

I go to Gillian's apartment and get a bunch of bananas. When I come back she is stable enough to transfer to the wards. Mr.

Wezzeh, Joseph, Gillian and I get her transferred to her bed and she woofs down four bananas and drinks some more water.

"I can eat rahce? I need so' rahce now!" she demands with a half smile and soon is in a well-deserved sleep.

Sketchy
August 21

Gillian asks me to round on pediatrics this morning. The hospital is filling back up again. The first patient I see on rounds is a two year old girl with an amulet around her neck.

"What is this?" I ask.

"Oh nuttin'," replies the mom with a sheepish grin.

"I have been in Africa for over 10 years. I know what this is and you know what it is."

"Somebody give it to huh to he'p huh."

"Yes, but what gives it its power? Is it God?"

"No."

"Then what? There are only two powers in this world...one of them is God and one is the enemy."

"It's nuttin'..."

"Every day, our staff prays for our patients, but if God answers our prayers and heals your daughter, will you thank him or will you think it is the amulet, charm, fetish, gris-gris?"

Everyone else in the room starts to laugh and chuckle. The mother looks even more sheepish and takes off the amulet and holds it in her hand.

"You should get rid of it, not just take it off..."

"I gonna gi' it to de man who gi' it to huh." Some battles aren't worth fighting. The baby is otherwise improving after Quinine and a blood transfusion. I move to the next patient.

"His stomach can huht him," says the mom.

"It takes malaria a few days to get better," I'm assuming he has malaria since he is on a Quinine drip. He was admitted yesterday by one of the PA's.

"He don' got malaria. His skin not hot. Yestuhdahy he take de whol' bottle o' medicine."

"Oh, really? What kind of medicine?"

"Blood tonic."
"What's that?"
"Medicine."
"Ok, can you bring it in so I can see it?"
"Yeah, no pwobluhm doctuh."

I stop the Quinine drip and move on. The boy looks stable anyway.

The next child is our little anemic boy who came in on death's door. I can barely recognize him now he looks so good. He still needs one more day of Quinine perfusion but he's definitely on the road to recovery.

Finally, I see baby Moses. Surprise, surprise, the urinary catheter came out. I repeat our daily ritual of cleaning it in diluted bleach and reinserting it. This time the bladder is not nearly so distended and the urine is pale and clear.

I go downstairs and start screening patients. A woman is brought in who looks very ill and is gurgling when she breathes.

"What's going on?" I ask the family.

"She tooth can huht huh an' now she ha' infekshuhn i' huh neck."

I examine her neck with a gloved hand and she does have a fluctuant area just under her mandible, suspicious for a well-developed abscess.

"Bring her in."

Otis and Phillip go get a wheelchair, wheel her into the exam room and put her on the table. R.B. from the ER starts an IV with a normal saline bolus and gives the antibiotic I ordered. I go up to the operating theater to get a scalpel, gloves, gauze and some lidocaine in a syringe.

Otis and Phillip then help me wheel/carry the girl up the stairs and then down to the pre-op room just in front of labor and delivery. I numb up the area over the abscess with difficulty as the woman jumps every time I prick her skin.

Once the local anesthetic is in, I incise down quickly. Thick, bloody pus wells out of the wound along with a clump of necrotic muscle. I stick in a gloved finger and sweep out some more dead flesh. She starts to really gurgle and yellow liquid pus starts pouring out her mouth.

"Get me a suction machine!"

Mr. Wezzeh brings in the suction machine and starts to aspirate out massive amounts of pus. I pack the neck wound and we send her to the wards.

Another patient is waiting in a car. The family states he has diabetes and slipped into a coma yesterday. They took him to the

ELWA hospital and was told he did not have Ebola. They present a handwritten note on a blank piece of paper stating he has "Diabetes: bad condition, septicemia, no suspicion of Ebola." Signed by the same Dr. Gunnar as the last slip of paper declaring a patient Ebola free. This time he's add: "MSF" (Médecins Sans Frontiers or Doctors Without Borders). It seems suspect to me.   ask if the patient is urinating frequently.

"No, no. He canno' pee pee free. Wuhn o' twoo tahms a day only."

I get more suspicious. I turn to examen the man. He's not breathing and has no pulse. Very sketchy. They want a death certificate. I state that I can't give it and I confiscate their "referral" slip. This needs to be followed up.

Is there really someone at the MSF Ebola treatment unit screening patients and writing on a hand written note that they are Ebola free without testing them? It's suspicious at best. I call Dr. Sonii. He agrees with me and says we will follow up in the morning.

I don't want to give them back the paper but they start to threaten. Dr. Sonii somehow gets word and calls me back.

"Bettuh to jus' make a copy an' give de papuh back to dem."

I'm learning that Dr. Sonii somehow always knows what's going on, even if he's not present. Maybe that's why he's always on the phone. I have Mitchell from accounting run out and make a photocopy. They will probably use the paper to get past police controls and bury him in a normal graveyard, exposing more people to the Ebola I suspect he died of. One of the lab techs, Jeff, calls the Ebola hotline and gives them the license plate of the car. The family takes the body away.

Bullet

August 22

I don't know if I'm just getting more stressed and sensitive (which is definitely true) or if everyone else is also really starting to feel the pressure. Patients seem more on edge, more pushy, more panicky.

As usual, I go outside the hospital early to screen patients. There are more and more of them everyday. As people have been afraid to come in to the hospital, they are waiting till the last minute and come in on death's door.

We have had many patients who are dead on arrival and many others who die shortly after admission. In all my 10 years in Africa I haven't seen death this frequently except the one Saturday back in Chad when there was a small war between the agriculturalists and the cattle herders. So many people here have severe hypertension, and at a young age. Strokes come in, several a day, and often in a coma. They usually die in a few days.

Now, people are impatient. They are clambering to be seen. They are annoyed and yelling, not the majority of course, but enough to set my already frayed nerves on edge. The security personnel, like Otis and Phillip, leave their posts on innocent missions and people take advantage to go in without washing their hands in chlorine water or being screened. Then when I try to get them to go back outside, some resist and argue. I can feel my stomach in a knot, squeezing and making it harder to breathe.

An ambulance pulls up. It's a mid-1990's Ford diesel van conversion, just like the two we have in Chad. The driver says they picked up a man who was walking in town and fell down with a grand mal seizure. As he's talking, the driver opens the back door to the ambulance. Inside are two EMTs covered from head to toe in protective gear, looking like they are about to handle radioactive material.

"What's happening?" I ask.
"He fell off an' seized. He got preshuh."
"What is his pressure?"
"Don' know."
"Do you have a blood pressure cuff?"
"No."

I go inside to the vital signs station and get a BP cuff from Bendu. I bring it outside and hand it to the men in the ambulance. They take the patient's blood pressure.

"Nothin'."
"What? His pressure is zero?"
"Yeah."
"Does he have a pulse? Is he breathing?"
They check. "No."
"Well he's dead then, take the body away."

They seem surprised and move quickly back away from the body. I fetch a basin of chlorine water.

"Put the stethoscope and BP cuff in here." They comply and begin talking agitatedly amongst themselves in Liberian English.

The driver grabs a bottle of some disinfectant solution and pours it over the two men's gloved and gowned hands. As I step back from the ambulance and look around I realize that all the patients that had been crowding around the entrance to the hospital have all pulled back. The crowd is now watching from a respectful distance. No one wants to come near. They all dread what I suspect the man died of: Ebola.

About 15 minutes after the ambulance leaves, I come back into the lobby from my office and am accosted by a belligerent man.

"Weh dey take de body o' de man in de ambulance? Gimme his numbuh."

"I don't have a number. And you need to go outside and not come in here without being screened."

He get's more insistent and finally I have to shout at him and almost forcefully expel him from the lobby. There are 2-3 others with him. They don't seem to get it that I don't have any info on who the ambulance people are. One of them shoots back a dirty look as he walks away from the door and shoots off some venomous words in my direction.

"Wha' you doin' heuh whahte man. Dis fo' de Liberians. Wha' you want heuh, huh?"

I start to sputter something off but everyone else around me is calming me, smiling and saying to just ignore him. I'm stressed out and my temper is on a short fuse. Things that normally would wash over me now seem like fighting words. I need a break. I go home and make myself some Ramon noodles. I chop up some tiny little eggplants called bitter balls and cook them with the noodles. I also add some dried fake meat. After eating, I pull back from the table with a sigh. I always feel better when I'm not hypoglycemic.

I go back out and there's another emergency "i' de cahr." I go outside and there are two cars waiting with patients inside.

"Who's first?" I ask.

Phillip points me to the car on my right. Inside is an elderly man in a coma with drool and froth coming out, gurgling when he breathes. I can guess what he has, but I ask anyway.

"What does he have?"

"Preshuh."

I knew it. I can't believe how severe hypertension is here. The story comes out that five days ago he couldn't move his left side. They didn't take him anywhere, afraid of going to a hospital with the Ebola epidemic going on. Yesterday, he stopped moving his right side and went into a coma.

I explain to the relatives gathered around that he's had a severe stroke. We could admit him but even if we were able to get his pressure down and he came out of his coma, he'd still be paralyzed. And he'd probably die a slow painful death due to aspiration, malnutrition and bedsores.

Here there aren't any rehab facilities for strokes. Anyway, considering his condition, he'd probably die in the hospital anyway like several others have already this week. I suggest they take him home. I give them a few minutes to think about it and go see the next patient.

"What's going on?" I inquire.

"He fine yestuhday. He feel tinglin' in his hans and take Ammo-die-a-quinn fo' de malaria. Today, he canna' eat, he can feel weak, reauhl weak."

"His skin can be hot? He throwin' out? Stomach running? Sore throat? Coughing? His hea' can huht him?" I try out my Liberian English on them and they mostly understand with a few puzzled glances among themselves. The reply is negative to all the screening questions.

I look at the patient. He's diaphoretic and cool to the touch of my gloved hand. He is semi-conscious and arousable. No staining anywhere to suggest incontinence, diarrhea or vomiting.

"He got shuguh," someone adds, meaning Diabetes.

I figure he's probably hypoglycemic from the Amodiaquine, probable malaria and not eating. I have them bring him in. R.B. and Habakuk quickly get an IV going and give him IV Dextrose. Jeff comes from the lab to draw his blood. Otis and Phillip take him up to the wards in a wheelchair via the staircase. The hospital has no elevator.

I go back to screening patients. A half hour later, Habakkuk comes from upstairs.

"De man throwin' out fast fast."

I go up and find the man I just admitted in his own room to the opposite side of the stairs from the other rooms. It turns out to be a fortuitous choice. I peer in the doorway. The man is lying on the ground, moving agitatedly, a pile of bilious vomit underneath him.

I get the family members some gloves and chlorine water to clean it up and go down to check on his labs. They are essentially normal except for "possibly" some malaria. Not likely to cause the man's severe symptoms in a hyper endemic area. I'm suspicious and feeling like I shouldn't have admitted him. Maybe it's early Ebola. Or the family was lying. I go back upstairs and find he has vomited two more times.

"Ok," I tell Alex and Habakuk. "We're shipping him out to the ELWA Hospital. He's got to go to the MSF treatment unit to get tested for Ebola."

I explain to the family that I suspect Ebola. They call a car while I get them protective gowns, gloves, masks, and hats. Then the four women (the male relatives have fled) carry the patient down to the car and we disinfect the room. I'm thankful that our staff are so careful in having as little contact as possible and wearing gowns, gloves, aprons and boots at all times.

I go downstairs and there's a young man named Titus lying in Paul's office. He was shot during the demonstration in West Point four day ago. Someone looted the Ebola isolation ward and all the patients fled. The bullet entered Titus' lower abdomen and there is no exit wound. He has been wandering from hospital to hospital, getting the occasional IV drip and wound dressing. None of the hospitals was willing to operate.

Finally, Titus went to the government hospital who brought him here. The surgeon requested to use our facilities so his team could do the operation here. Fortunately, our administrator, Mrs. Carter, is a strong woman and a straight shooter. She told them no way. We have our own surgeons and they have their own well stocked facility. Either they operate on him at their hospital or we operate on him here. Period. They left dropped Titus off and left.

Amazingly, Titus is able to walk upstairs to the theater with almost no assistance. The anesthetist hasn't showed, so I offer to do anesthesia for Gillian. I give him a spinal and Gillian starts the operation. The spinal doesn't anesthetize the upper abdomen. When Gillian starts exploring the upper quadrants, Titus starts flinching. I inject 10mg of Diazepam and 100mg of Ketamine. Then I start a Ketamine drip through one of his IV lines.

Gillian finds four holes in the small bowel and one in the rectum. Amazingly, after four days, his abdomen isn't full of stool or pus. He's managed to wall off the stool in the left lower quadrant which is certainly why he's still alive today.

Gillian inserts a suction catheter into the first hole in the bowel to clean it out. The suction tip gets clogged and when she pulls it out there's a four inch long round worm attached and still wiggling! She completes the rest of the four hour operation, doing a bowel resection, side to side anastamosis, rectum repair and colostomy.

When Gillian starts to put the edematous intestines back inside the abdominal cavity, Titus starts to vomit. So much for the NG tube which is supposed to empty his stomach! I call for suction, but we only have one machine. Joseph detaches Gillian's tubing and then attaches another one for me.

Finally, I am able to suction out the green goo gurgling out his mouth as he desaturates into the 60's. The first thing I pull out is another four inch long round worm, also squirming and curling. I clear out the rest of the gunk and Gillian finishes the case.

He is having a harder time keeping his sats up after vomiting. I'm afraid he's aspirated. With a lot of oxygen his O2 sats are staying the low normal range. However, prior to throwing up, Titus' sats were 100% on 2L of oxygen. I listen to his lungs as Mr. Wezzeh dresses the wounds and drains.

I notice he has markedly diminished sounds on the right. I percuss and find dullness to percussion. I know it might be fluid in the lung from aspiration, but don't want to miss something else since we don't have x-ray. I take a sterile 5cc syringe and carefully insert it above one of the anterior ribs. Just posterior to the rib I get a sudden flush back of liquid mixed with blood.

Gillian puts in a chest tube and his breathing improves. Actually, she puts in a large foley catheter since we don't have any chest tubes. But is seems to be working. Joseph and Mr. Wezzeh wheel Titus out to the ward as soon as he starts to move and come out of his anesthesia.

He leaves with quite the collection of paraphernalia: an NG tube, a chest tube, two IVs, a surgical drain, a colostomy bag and a urinary catheter. Alex and Habakkuk tie him to the bed to make sure he doesn't pull anything out since he might get agitated when coming off the Ketamine. I go home exhausted and hypoglycemic. It's after 10:00PM. I make myself two peanut butter sandwiches, prostrate myself, pray, cry a lot and go to bed.

Death
August 24

Gillian's taking the day off. She hasn't had one in a long time. I start with rounds on the inpatient ward. One of the first patients I see doesn't look so good. She came in for an incomplete spontaneous abortion and had a D&C two days ago. She's not bleeding now, but had severe anemia. Unfortunately, she was only transfused one unit of blood.

We have no blood bank and depend on family members to donate. No one has come for her. She's breathing shallow and fast, but is awake and alert. She complains of upper abdominal pain. I put on gloves and palpate an enormous, tender liver extending all the way down to her belly button. Not a good sign. She's already on Malaria treatment. I add an antibiotic to cover typhoid and continue the IV fluids. I encourage her to drink a lot of water.

There are 24 patients on the inpatient service. Many of the postpartum women I send home, including the Muslim woman who just delivered twins yesterday morning. She gets her shot of anti-D Immunoglobulin. Her blood type is O-. She thanks me profusely, as does her husband. "Al hamdullilah!" I say, much to their surprise and pleasure.

I also send home the young boy who had come in Thursday nearly dead of severe malaria and anemia. He is now fully active and eating without fever or anemia. Little Moses is still hanging around to get his bladder intermittently catheterized since we have no balloon catheters small enough for his premie size urethra.

I spend time with a fat hypertensive Muslim man with malaria. I explain how he can control and even cure his "preshuh" with diet. He is very receptive. "As salaam alekum," I say in parting as the reply echoes in my ears "…wa alekum as salaam!"

Titus is doing better two days post-op, except for periodically pulling on his tubes. Today, he's disconnected his chest tube from the water seal again. I reinsert it the tube in the bottle of water and try to reason with him. Otherwise, he is improving nicely. He has clear drainage from his abdominal drain, but no air or stool in his colostomy bag yet.

I go down to my office. Dr. Sonii passes by and we discuss how to stream line the Ebola screening process for new patients. I suggest that it should be the PA's that screen. Dr. Sonii calls in Timothy, the PA on duty, and he quickly grasps the idea. We give him a new toy we just got: an infrared thermometer allowing us to check for fever without touching the patient. Very useful in the Ebola capital of the world.

I go for lunch. As I finish eating, I get a phone call from Alex, "The patient in M1 is not doing well."

I go upstairs to the wards. The patient with hepatomegaly is barely breathing and unconscious. Her pulse is rapid and thready. I open up the IV running with Saline and give her some D50 in case she has hypoglycemia (we have no way of testing). I ask Alex to start another IV which he does quickly. I raise the IV pole so the fluids can go in rapidly and raise her legs to drain blood to her head and vital organs.

She starts to wake up, mumbles some words, moves around and then stops breathing. I check her pulse. Nothing. I don't bother with CPR since I know that what she needs is a blood transfusion. Since there's none available, resuscitation is useless. Plus, her enlarged liver means many of her other vital organs are probably shut down. I shake my head and offer my condolences to her sister standing beside her. Then I walk out.

Bendu calls me downstairs to see two patients just arrived by personal auto. The first is a sickle cell patient with severe anemia. He'd been treated for malaria four days ago with three days of Artemether injections. This continues to affirm my suspicion that Artemether is almost completely useless as a malaria treatment.

His dad noticed he was very pale today, called his regular doctor at the ELWA Hospital. The doctor told him they didn't have the supplies to do blood transfusions and referred him to Dr. Martin, our other staff physician. Dr. Martin told them he was in a meeting and to come see me.

The boy is 17 years old, thin and very pale all over. He is very weak, breathing shallow and semi-conscious. My heart sinks. But I have to try. Otis and Phillip help me bring him into the consultation room in a wheelchair. I call Jeff to see if he can come in from home. He says he'll be right there.

I go to see the patient in the other car. She has "preshuh" and has been feeling "weeeak!" for two days. She is unconscious, but the family denies any other symptoms, including fever. I check her mouth and eyes with a gloved hand for signs of bleeding. There are none. I feel her forehead and it feels hot. I take her temperature: 101.7. I refer her to the ELWA Hospital for Ebola testing. She's 74 years old and has already had a previous stroke. She's not going to make it, Ebola or not.

I go back inside the hospital. The father of the sickle cell anemia patient calls me over.

"What happenin'? He convuhsing?"

I go in to the exam room and find the boy almost dead. There is an occasional agonal gasp, but he's completely unconscious.

"He's dying…" I blurt.

As the father panics, I put my finger on the boy's carotid pulse, it's still strong initially, but quickly disappears under my touch as he stops breathing completely.

"I'm sorry, he's passed…" I gently inform the distraught father.

"No, no, don' leave me…after all dis…no, no, no!" I turn away, my heart broken by this man's sorrow and loss, but feeling helpless at the same time.

R.B. comes to me five minutes later and says there are fluids coming out of the boy. I look in the room and he has urinated all over the floor, as happens often after death when everything relaxes. But R.B is a little worried. Ebola is on everyone's mind and we all have a healthy fear of bodily fluids now.

I go get some full body isolation suits, one for Otis and another for me. We gown and glove up and wheel the body out to the waiting Toyota Forerunner. We dump the body unceremoniously in the back, not bothering to arrange it since we want as little contact as possible, even with our yellow and white full body jumpsuits. I take a final look at the floppy body, legs sprawled at weird angles and head bent to allow the back door to close…then I slam it shut.

I remove my suit. Otis removes his. We put them in a red, biohazard bag and Otis takes it out back to the incinerator to burn it. The cleaning team is already spraying everything down with chlorine water and cleaning up.

I go upstairs. I've just come from checking on three patients apparently I'd missed during morning rounds when Habakuk comes up excitedly saying "De President comin'! De President comin'!"

For reasons unknown to me, she is coming to see Titus. Dark suited, large men come up first and take up security positions. Then an entourage of equally dark-suited men and smartly dressed women come up. In the middle is a middle aged woman with gray hair, walking confidently with a straight back, wearing blue jeans and a sweater. It's obvious by the looks and mannerisms of all around that this is the Ellen Johnson Sirleaf, the President of Liberia.

Mrs. Carter, our administrator, introduces me and we walk down to see Titus. The President asks me how Titus is doing. I give her an update and then she spends a long time talking with the young man's grandmother. Then she thanks the staff and walks out, chatting with Mrs. Carter. Mrs. Carter has taken the initiative to ask for government help in procuring some of the supplies we need desperately in order to stay open. The President thanks us for staying open during the crises, gives US$ 200 to the nurses on duty and encourages us to continue our work.

I go home, eat leftover rice and curry and crash into bed.

Pit
August 25

Today is a holiday in Liberia. Not that anyone feels like celebrating much with the Ebola crisis projected to last 6-9 more months. As Mitchell from accounting tells me later when I ask how was his holiday:

"Boring. We canno' do anyting. Everyone 'fraid to go out. Before we use ta go see friends, ha' some ice cream, but wid dis Ebola ting, we 'fraid to go out."

Mitchell really wants me to go see his family out in their village. His father is 99 years old and has been blind since the '70s. According to the legend, he was out working in his fields and lay down to take a nap. An enemy came and sprinkled a special dust in his eyes and he went blind despite trying all the leaves, roots, potions, charms, fetishes and witchcraft available. He still is strong, otherwise. They have rigged a system of guide ropes around the compound so he can get from place to place. And he still rules the roost.

On this holiday morning, I oversleep. I'm exhausted. Gillian has mostly finished rounds when I get up to the floor. I go see Mr. Carter, the husband of our administrator. He has not improved. When I look at the chart, he has only received one of the six bottles of IV fluids he should have received since admission yesterday. And his quinine was only given twice instead of three times. I call Philip, the veteran nurse on duty (not to be confused with Phillip the security guard). He quickly starts another IV and tries to make up for lost time.

Dede comes up to talk to me about a patient who has been in active labor since yesterday. The midwife on duty yesterday didn't inform either Gillian or I that the patient wasn't progressing. She is now at only 5cm but has just broken her bag of water. I tell Dede we will see if this spontaneous rupture of membranes can get things going and tell her to inform me if there is no cervical change in the next couple hours.

Gillian has found a surfboard for me. Her friend, Pete, had an extra one. He prefers to Stand Up Paddle surf anyway. We make lunch and get ready to go to the beach. The sun is finally shining, but there is some wind. We'll see how the surf is. Just then Dede comes to see me.

"De fetal hahht rate 168 per minute."

"That's ok, as long as it doesn't go low."

"She not progressin'. doc. You shoul' come see huh."

"Ok." I follow Dede up the two flights of stairs and then down the stairs from the wards into the labor and delivery suite next to the theater.

I check the woman and she is dilated at 7-8 cm. Dede points to the partograph:

"Intuhvenshun," she states matter of factly. I really don't want to do a c-section.

"How are her contractions?"

"Good, doc."

I put my hand on the patient's abdomen. She is having regular contractions but not very strong enough. They are short lived, lasting only 10-15 seconds.

"Let's start her on Pit," I say. "Put 20 units of Oxytocin in 500ml of RL."

Dede sets up the drip. I start it slow and continue to monitor the woman's contractions with my hand on her belly. Within a few minutes the contractions are getting stronger and lasting longer. There's still with good relaxation in between the contractions. Within 15 minutes the woman exclaims:

"I gotta toilet!"

I check her and the infant's head has come down. She is now completely dilated except for an anterior cervical lip that I reduce manually with the next contraction. She starts pushing and in another 15 minutes has delivered a strong boy screaming his lungs out.

I wash up and head home. We get in the Gillian's car with her "adopted" baby. He was premature and the mother initially abandoned him for several days. Gillian cared for him and then the mother came back. Gillian maintains contact with the mother and baby and takes him from time to time. She's had him since yesterday.

We drive down the main highway in Monrovia which parallels the beach. We have been told there is surf at "A La Lagune" resort.

Ebola-iculous

We follow the signs but find, not surprisingly, a lagoon with no way to the beach.

We ask for directions to the beach and follow a dirt road to a cement block making business right on the beach. Trash is piled high and I have to pick my way through a swamp and garbage to a rocky beach with a tiny stretch of sand. Plastic waste is strewn everywhere and a young child is just finishing depositing a poop log worthy of a much larger man. The waves are crazy! A huge swell tossed and turned by a fierce wind has created a turbulent chop that is positively frightening.

We go back to the main road and drive south towards the airport. Gillian says there's supposed to be another good spot near a resort that begins with a "K". I see a sign that might be something so we turn down a paved road that ends on the beach near a nice hotel.

The sand is clean and the waves are still crazy even here. But I'm desperate to surf. I walk down the beach and choose a place where the angle of the land makes the waves come in not too strong. I paddle out. It's intimidating going up and down and sideways over these huge, choppy swells.

Finally, I'm out a long ways from shore. I paddle over to where the waves are breaking. A huge wave piles above me. I turn and paddle and get caught by a huge surge. I get to my feet but there is no wax on the board and my front foot slips off. I get tumbled a bit and get back on just in time to catch the next wave. Each wave breaks and reforms three times before hitting the beach. I catch the next two sections in and jump off right on the beach.

I'm done.

Sudden

August 26

The man is complaining of abdominal pain, just like pretty much everyone who comes in to the hospital. I often don't even examine them. For some reason, this time, I put on gloves and have him get up on the exam table. He has a palpable mass in the upper center of his abdomen. I order an ultrasound.

After the man pays, I take him into Dr. Martin's office and ask him if he'll do the scan. He pleasantly agrees. A few minutes later he comes out and gets me to come in. He shows me a well-circumscribed lesion with fluid in it.

"He has an amebic liver abscess here in de left lobe," Dr. Martin moves the probe around and I clearly see normal liver and then another, smaller fluid collection. "Here a second, smaller one in de right lobe."

Dr. Martin goes to look for a large bore spinal needle, a syringe and a few other things to drain the large abscess using the ultrasound as a guide. He comes back and hasn't been able to locate a large bore spinal needle. We decide to hospitalize him, put him on IV Flagyl to treat the amebas. We'll try again tomorrow when staff are around to help us find the materials we need.

The next day is really busy with lots of OB patients and lots of out-patients. Dr. Martin does a c-section. As a result, it's not until the evening that Gillian has a chance to go drain the man's liver abscess. I'm making supper when she comes back.

"That's not a liver abscess! That's a huge abdominal aortic aneurysm!"

"Are you sure? I swore I saw a liver abscess."

"Let's go look."

"Yeah. Let's."

We go up to the wards. I take the ultrasound and place it on the man's abdomen. Now it seems obvious that the mass isn't in the liver but is rather an enlarged, calcified, pulsating mass otherwise known as an abdominal aortic aneurysm. It extends into the thorax. Not good. There's no hospital in Liberia equipped to do the surgery he needs. The closest possible place, according to Gillian, is probably Nigeria. Not that they really want to take anyone from Liberia since it was a Liberian who brought Ebola to Nigeria.

We explain the situation to the patient and he assures us his employers will be able to arrange things. We tell him to try and relax and we go back to eat supper.

After supper, I go to write emails and Skype with my family. Dede pokes her head in my office door.

"De patient in N3 goin' into shock."

I'm trying to think which OB patient it could be since Dede's a midwife. I arrive at the door of room N3 and see it's our patient with the aneurysm. He is contorting in pain, his legs lifted high up in the air. He's rocking back and forth. In between moans he manages to blurt out a dire prediction:

"I gonna die! I gonna die!"

I try to calm him down as I ask the nurses to bring some Diazepam. Getting anxious and increasing his blood pressure will not be good for his aneurysm.

"What is his blood pressure?"

"It wa' 160/100, den it quickly drop ta 80/40 and now I don' find anyting, doc," says Alex calmly, dressed in green scrubs and plastic apron, looking up with a stethoscope still in his ears and the hand pump on the blood pressure cuff still in his hand.

I feel the man's carotid pulse...nothing. He's gasping for air. The gasps get less and less frequent as his contortions slow and then stop. His aneurysm has burst, causing him to bleed out in a matter of minutes right before our eyes. It's an eery and helpless feeling. He has no family with him. One of the nurses takes his cell phone and starts calling numbers trying to find a relative.

I pull of my gloves, snap them into the trash can and go home. The body is gone in the morning.

Eyes
August 27

    I can start to see it in their eyes. They just have that look. Maybe I'm starting to imagine things in my paranoia, but I'm beginning to think I can recognize an Ebola patient on sight. Maybe it's my intuition. Maybe it's that still small voice I've been praying helps me out. Maybe I'm imagining it.

    The eyes kind of bulge out. They have a sort of blank stare. The inside of the eyelids are more red than normal. The surface of the eyes, the white part, the scleral conjunctiva seems to be a little edematous and not quite the right color: not quite yellow as in jaundice, but not quite white either. It's subtle.

    Ambulances are starting to pull up more regularly. I get called outside and find the first ambulance with it's back towards me, doors swung open and a well dressed man with some kind of badge inside telling me to come and look. I first find the ambulance driver, the same one who brought the already dead body the other day.

"He's alive this time, right?"

The driver laughs nervously, and nods. I turn to the heavyset woman who seems to be the spokesperson for the family.

"What's happening?"

"He walkin' along an' he jus' start cohnvuhsing. He bahte hi' tongue and hi' arm shakin' like dis." She gives me a visual of arms pumping up and down.

"How long did it last?"

"An hour."

"Did he come to…was he conscious afterwards, or sleepy?"

"He didna wake up."

    I climb up the rear step of the ambulance and gingerly crawl in, trying not to touch anything. With my gloved hand I pull down his eyelid. He has a blank stare and is in a coma. I can't see his pupils, it's too dark inside the ambulance. His eyes seem slightly edematous. I open his mouth. All his teeth and tongue are covered with old and new blood. It gives me a start, like catching the look of a hyena in your spotlight as he lifts his bloody mouth from his prey and laughs at you. I instinctively pull back. I back pedal quickly out of the ambulance.

"You're not telling me the full truth," I inform the large woman and the well-dressed man as I peel off my gloves and go to wash my hands and arms in chlorine water. "Take him to EWLA Hospital to see Doctors Without Borders. He needs to be tested for Ebola."

I go inside to check on the two patients I've admitted earlier. One elderly man is having an acute exacerbation of his heart failure. His lung bases are filled with fluid and his lower legs are tense and shiny with pitting edema. He has gotten his first dose of Lasix, but the foley hasn't been placed yet. It's Philip again, the nurse who didn't give most of the medicine to our administrator's husband the first day he was hospitalized. I go off on him and he scurries to put in the foley and reports back to me that there is 700mL in the bag.

The second man has probably been having a heart attack for the last three days. It certainly sounds like typical chest pain which now occurs even at rest. I gave him an aspirin when he walked in the door. Without an EKG or any other way to diagnose or treat a heart attack definitively, I admit him for accelerated medical management. His pain is a little better after a shot of Pentazocine, the closest thing we have to morphine.

I go back downstairs and the ambulance is still there and the fat woman and distinguished man are inside. I'm getting the idea the man thinks that just because he's someone important he can make us take this patient. I ask them to please go outside. There is resistance but I insist and finally they grudgingly go outside. The man is obviously upset, muttering something about being in law enforcement or something. I have to stand at the door and keep insisting before they finally drive off.

Paul, the PA, is falling behind in the screening process. There is a crowd inside that's already been screened, but another, even larger crowd waits outside. I start helping him screen patients. Mrs. Wennie motions me over into her office with her hand.

"Can I speak wit' you a minute, doctuh?" I go into her office, right next to the outpatient pharmacy.

"Yeah, what is it?"

She shows me a slip of paper with a last name and then two different first names separated by an "or". Underneath is written "yellow shirt, black jacket and blue jeans".

"Dat man sittin' outside, over der..." She points to the right side of the courtyard. "...someone call and tell me he suspicious for Ebola. One o' his relatives die o' Ebola."

I go out and ask the man some questions. It sounds like he has malaria. He doesn't look sick. But it could be early Ebola. I prescribe him some medicine, find out how much it will cost and take his US$ 15 inside to pay for his consultation fee and meds. I bring them out to him, explain how to take them and then warn him if he doesn't get better in a couple days to go get tested for Ebola.

After lunch and some more screening, I start to consult patients. Dr. Martin is falling behind due to the sheer number of cases. I see a young boy with a hernia and a middle aged man with a huge inguinal scrotal hernia. I schedule both for surgery tomorrow.

I'm up on the wards, seeing how the two patients I admitted earlier are doing. The man with heart failure has now put out a total of 1900mL of clear urine after two doses of Lasix. The man with chest pain is lying comfortably in bed. I go to the nurses station to talk to Philip and we hear another ambulance pull up. I go downstairs to investigate.

This ambulance is parked parallel to the hospital with the side doors open. The patient is sitting in the paramedic's chair. He quickly gets up and drops his pants to show me why he came. There is a large mass in his right scrotum extending up into his inguinal canal.

He states it came out earlier today and is getting more painful. He vomited once. No fever or diarrhea or other problems. I have him come in the hospital. I call down Philip and Gillian comes as well. Habakuk helps Philip start an IV while Gillian dons gloves and starts gently squeezing the mass. She wants to get the air out of the intestines so the hernia will reduce.

I give the man Diazepam and Ketamine to help him relax and to relieve his pain. Instead, he tenses up, his arms rigid, in a typical Ketamine reaction. I give him more Valium and he relaxes just as Gillian pops the intestines back inside the abdomen. He has no one with him and is out cold from the meds. We leave him in the exam room, hoping family will show up or that he can contact someone when he wakes up.

Gillian meanwhile has gone out to see another patient. I'm sitting in my office when she walks in.

"I'd like you to see this patient. The woman says she is six months pregnant and doesn't feel the baby move. She had fever, diarrhea and vomiting yesterday but none today. Her conjunctiva are very red though. Supposedly she got 5 days of malaria treatment already and her normal hospital, JFK, refused her because they don't take patients at night."

I go out and look in the back seat of the car. The woman is semiconscious, her eyes kind of swollen with an abnormal color to the white part. I peel down her eyelid and the conjunctiva are really, really red. I suddenly get inspiration.

"How many times did you toilet today?"

"Two times."

"How many times did you vomit today?"

"Four times."

I turn to the family, "She is very suspicious for Ebola. We cannot take her. She needs to go to the EWLA Hospital and see Doctors Without Borders to get tested for Ebola."

The woman next to the patient speaks up "But she pregnant... she don' ha' Ebola..."

"Pregnancy is not a vaccine against Ebola. She needs to be tested. We cannot take her." And I walk away.

No Blood
August 30

I'm outside in Gillian's car by 5:50AM, waiting for the curfew to lift. At 6:00AM sharp, I start racing through the streets of Monrovia to Oddny Beach. The surf is still big and rough. I can't even get past the break. After finally succumbing to exhaustion, I catch some white water to go in. It forms back up and allows me a few brief seconds of actual stand up surfing before I'm back on the beach.

Just as I get back to the car, I get a call from the nursing station saying that the patient with alcohol withdrawal syndrome just passed. Alex states it in traditional Liberian nursing code:

"De man got no vital signs."

I travel the 20 minutes back to the SDA Cooper Hospital. I park in front of the gate to the hospital compound. I turn off the car and walk towards the main entrance. I need to go through the hospital and open the gate from the inside. see the young man who's been staying with Mrs. Carter's husband while he's been hospitalized this last week.

"Morning, how is it?" I ask.

"Fine," he says with a half smile.

I walk past but hear another voice behind me.

"Doctuh…" I turn and see another relative of Mrs. Carter's getting out of the car I just walked past.

"Yes…?"

"I jus' wanna tank you fo' yo' efforts for de ol' man."

"Ok, no problem…" Mr. Carter must've died overnight. I confirm it up at the nursing station in a couple minutes.

I go open the gate and bring in the car. I open my apartment, take a cold bucket shower and go into the hospital. As I open the door to my office I see another young man. He's been faithfully by the side of his aging diabetic father who came in with severe anemia and cerebral malaria. We'd transfused him several times and had been treating him for several days with not much improvement. The young man stops me.

"Tanks, doc, yo' done yo' best fo' ma fadduh. It wa' jus' his tahme. Tanks fo' everyting…" And I know he would've shaken my hand if Ebola hadn't made that ancient ritual suddenly obsolete.

Death continues to stalk us, and it's not just Ebola. Many patients wait till the last minute to come in to get treated because of the fear they might catch Ebola in the hospital. Yet, in spite of it all, the thankful, generous spirit of the Liberians shines through.

An hour or so later, I'm sitting in church. We've just finished the Bible Study. Now the choir is warming up the crowd. It's Women's Ministries weekend and the ladies are taking charge with enthusiasm. The choir sways down the aisles singing a song of welcome as they march up to the raised choir loft about 20 feet above where I'm sitting.

The service moves along with many selections by the all female choir. On the platform, it's all women. A lady has just finished giving her testimony.

She fled Liberia to Ivory Coast during the war. She swore she was going to learn French, change her citizenship and never go back to Liberia. Then, a friend called and asked her to come help them with a new organization. Some Liberians were forming this agency to help the female child soldiers recover from their many traumas after the war finished. She prayed about it and came back. She has been helping women and children suffering from violence and abuse in her organization's safe house ever since.

The choir is just about to let it rip again when I hear an ambulance on the street outside. I have a feeling about where it's going. I pull my phone out of my pocket in anticipation of the call I expect to come. Sure enough, in the middle of the choir's number, I get a call. I quickly leave my front row seat, duck under the bar across the open door and go outside. I can barely hear over the roar of the church's generator, but I do catch the word "emerjuhcee".

"I'll be right there," I reply. I walk around the corner and up the half block to the Cooper SDA Hospital.

An ambulance is outside the main doors. Inside is a boy about 10 years old who's actively seizing. I ask a couple of brief questions.

"He got no blood," reply the anxious parents.

I verify by looking at his white palpebral conjunctiva, "Bring the child in."

I call for a nurse from the inpatient ward since outpatient is closed on Saturdays. It's Alex and he quickly establishes an IV. I give the boy some glucose and then a loading dose of Quinine in a drip.

Alex gives him the Artemether in his thigh muscle. He then injects an antibiotic. Fortunately, Jeff is here. I have him do a hemoglobin and type and cross for a blood transfusion. The boy is still seizing. I ask Alex to get me some Diazepam. I inject the drug in small increments until I've given him 20mg, enough to knock me out for days! Finally, he stops convulsing. Luckily he's also still breathing.

Jeff soon comes with the results: his hemoglobin is 3! The good news is that his older brother also has O+ blood and is willing to donate. Unfortunately, Jeff only fills the adult blood bag about ½ full. I come in just in time to see him finishing up. I tell him to fill up another pediatric bag from the brother. That way the kid will get a full adult bag dose of 450ml. It turns out to be a good thing that the blood is donated in two separate bags.

Otis calls me to see another child. This one is four years old and also has "no blood." He is floppy, and appears to be intermittently seizing as well. The mom has put a tongue depressor wrapped in gauze between his teeth to keep him from biting his tongue. He looks like death warmed over.

The mom is sweetly singing songs about Jesus as she intermittently prays in a loud voice, "Jeeesus! Jeeesus! JEEEEEESUS!"

We get an IV in the child, start the Quinine drip, give him an Artemether shot and have Jeff type and cross match his blood. He also has O+. He looks like he may die any second now. We really don't have time to test the child's young father.

I grab the second bag of blood still waiting for the first child. I bring it to the ER and have Alex hook it up to the kid's IV line. The family can replace it later with another donor. Alex takes him upstairs 15 minutes later. He is already breathing easier and opening his eyes. He is no longer seizing. Blood is a wonderful thing.

The first kid, though, continues to intermittently convulse. I keep giving him Diazepam. We keep him in the ER.

Another boy comes in referred from an outside clinic. They did a hemoglobin since he had "no blood" and found it to be a little over 5. He seems alert, though, and not too pale. I start a quinine drip, give Artemether and send him upstairs. Jeff has left already and won't be back until the evening. At 5:00PM Jeff is back and confirms that boy's hemoglobin is 7. We don't transfuse.

Meanwhile, the next bag of blood is ready for our first kid. He's still occasionally seizing. I get the transfusion running and send him upstairs. I have Alex give him some more Diazepam. In less than 12 hours he's gotten over 50mg of Diazepam, enough to stop me breathing for sure. He still isn't completely convulsion free. I hear the mom talking to a relative on the phone:

"I pu' my faif i Gawd…" That's all we can do sometimes.

Later that evening, I check up on the Pediatric ward. A girl admitted yesterday with "no blood" and a hemoglobin of 2.3 is lying comfortably in her bed. She's been awake and eating all day, looking again like the cute little girl she is. Her second transfusion is running. The first one only got her hemoglobin up to 5. Her mother is just finishing up her prayers, bowing towards Mecca. She gets up, looks at her daughter and smiles.

"As salaam aleikum," I say as I smile back.

Scars

September 1

A large Muslim woman with a head scarf and long sleeved dress with Middle Eastern patterned embroidery comes into my office. I can tell she is nervous. I've sent her to be tested because she is the third wife of a man I just tested and found to be HIV+.

She sits in the chair across the desk, her hands folded in her lap as she anxiously bites her lower lip.

"I have your test results and the HIV test is negative."

The woman starts to cry and wail.

"Jus' counsel me, doctuh…tell me de truhf."

"Ma'am, calm down. You don't have HIV…"

She falls off the chair and starts writhing on the ground wailing. She looks up at me with bleary eyes as tears roll down her cheeks.

"Oh! Oh! OH!" She slowly pulls herself together and sits back on the chair.

"Ma'am I don't think you understood. The test is ok, it's good. You don't have the disease…"

"Oh tank God. Tank God. Look at dis…" And she lifts up her sleeve to reveal scars on her forearm and a massive, stellate scar on the back of her upper arm.

"I a war victim. Dey torture' me. I shounnah be alive. Look at dis…"

She lifts up her skirt and shows me an equally enormous scar on her thigh. She raises her hands and eyes to heaven.

"God is great! I not wanna marry dis man. My mudduh force me. He own many stores, he rich. He take care of my mudduh and brudduh. I ha' no fadduh. But I de tird wife o' dis man. I knew it wasna mah destiny."

She falls on her face on the ground reciting some words in Arabic "Allahu Akbar…la ila illa Al-Lah" then she gets up.

"I knew when they wan' a take ma blood. I knew the test woul' be positive o' negative. So I went to pray and I pray to God. Now I know God love me. I know he love me. I will be free." And she continues to cry.

I'm not sure what to say, so I don't say anything.

"Tank you, doctuh and tank God. He has saved me. I will go back to ma family now. He save me fra' de war and He save me fra' dis disease. Allahu akbar. Doctuh, may God protect you and not let anyting' hurt you. All dis Ebola, may God not let it near you. Tank you. You ha' been straight wid me. I know God loves me."

As she walks out I call out to her, "As salaam aleikum…"

She turns and smiles, "Wa aleikum as salaam doctuh."

Ebola-iculous

September 2

I've been seeing so many kids with severe malaria and anemia that I let my guard down. Because of the Ebola epidemic, parents are waiting till the last minute to bring in their children. Fortunately, so far we've been able to save most of them with blood transfusions and Quinine drips.

As a result, when I go out to see this 10 year old girl, in my mind I've already decided she has malaria. I go through the motions of asking all the screening questions and she sounds like she has malaria: headache, fever, loss of appetite, no vomiting or diarrhea.

Instinctively, I check her eyelids to see if she has anemia like everyone else. Most of the kids have had very pale palpebral conjunctiva, but this girl's are bright red. It sets of warning bells in my head, but I ignore my instinct. It's probably malaria I tell myself. I don't want to send her to certain death from malaria by refusing her. I let her come in the hospital against my gut feeling.

I hope the mistake doesn't turn out to be too costly.

I bring her into the ER and R.B. finds an IV. As she is taping the catheter in place she asks me if I've noticed the rash. The girl has a raised rash all over her arms and trunk and face. It doesn't look like anything I've seen before.

I've just given her an Artemether shot in her muscle. There was no bleeding. Now I look back and some blood is pooling over the injection site. Jeff from the lab is right there. I ask him to go get a rapid malaria test and do it here at bedside. Meanwhile, R.B. starts the Quinine drip.

I look again at the child's conjunctiva. They really are more red then normal! I'm starting to get a suspicious feeling. Sure enough, the malaria smear is normal. Where Jeff pricked her finger is also bleeding more than normal. And she has a high fever. There's a reason they call it Ebola Hemorrhagic fever. Of all the suspicious cases we've had here, this is the first one I've seen with bleeding. This is definitely the most suspicious case for Ebola I've seen yet.

I call in the mother. She's dressed in some kind of police or security uniform. I explain that I'm suspicious of Ebola and they should take her immediately to either of the Ebola Treatment Units: the JFK government hospital or the EWLA Hospital where Doctors Without Borders has set up shop.

They leave immediately. We wash down everything and throw away anything that we may have touched with our contaminated gloves. I run home, take a shower, wash my scrubs in disinfectant and put on new clothes. I feel this is my closest contact with Ebola yet.

A few hours later, the mother is back with the girl in the back of a car.

"Dey look at de IV and say to take her back to where she bein' treated…"

Are you kidding me!? It turns out that neither Treatment Unit would take her. Both are overrun. Dr. Martin comes out and tries to call some colleagues who work at JFK. No one is picking up. There just aren't enough isolation beds or tents or personnel or supplies or anything. They are turning away patients left and right. But to not even test? And to use the excuse that she is being treated elsewhere to turn her away? And all because we left the IV in to help them out so they could treat her without the risks of starting another IV?

I admit, some NON-MISSIONARY WORDS not only come to mind, but a few slip out at high volume. They seem the only words worthy of expressing my feelings about the ridiculousness of the situation.

I do what I should've done before: I write out a referral explaining why we think she has Ebola. I tell them to go back and don't let themselves be turned away. Dr. Martin also suggests a third hospital, Redemption which is supposed to be opening—and we hope is already open—as an Ebola Treatment Unit.

Obviously—and rightfully so—the family is frustrated and turns away sorrowfully. Who knows? No one probably ever will. She will probably die without us ever knowing if she had Ebola or some treatable disease.

If there were only the resources available to isolate all the suspicious cases and test them. Then if they are negative, get them referred to a hospital such as our own which is treating non-Ebola cases. And if they have Ebola, there should be personnel, protective gear and IV fluids to treat them.

Instead, chaos, fear, suspicion, lies and death abounds in the Ebola Capital of the World.

Interrogation
September 3

I feel like I'm in a bad movie.

I've been called over by the Department of Defense to testify. A uniformed woman leads the way in her SUV as the hospital's van transports Dr. Sonii and I to the walled compound of the Armed Forces of Liberia. We get out in the rain, walk past a seriously black and shiny SUV, enter the lobby and march past the camouflaged guards.

We continue down a couple hallways, past large photos of soldiers doing humanitarian tasks like helping out in schools and battling floods and up to a double door with a full length mirror to the right. Above the mirror it says "watch your uniform". Our escort pauses briefly to make sure her uniform is up to standard. Then we walk in. I'm more than a little embarrassed in my jeans and t-shirt, which is the best clothes I brought to Liberia.

A tall man with a big smile welcomes us and asks us to take a seat. The rest of the men in the room are more somber and intimidating. The man, who appears to be the head of the commission, informs me that they'd like me to give a statement about the patient we operated on a few Fridays ago with the alleged gun shot wound.

Dr. Sonii is escorted out. I'm called to come to the middle of the U-shaped formation of tables. There is a single chair there facing the chief. He is flanked by two other well-dressed men not in uniform.

The head of the commission asks me to take an oath. I agree and am motioned over to my left where lay a Bible, a Qur'an and another book I don't take the time to identify. I'm asked to choose which I would like to swear on. I briefly think of the Qur'an but place my hand on the Bible instead. I'm informed I can pick it up if I want to. The way it's said makes me want to, so I do.

The classic formula of "I swear to tell the truth, the whole truth and nothing but the truth so help me God" is read out to me in brief spurts which I am told to repeat. I meekly comply. I put the Bible down and return to my small chair in the midst of important men.

The chief instructs me to begin my statement. I describe first meeting Titus. I explain what kind of exam I did. I give the details of the surgery, as I saw them, from the head of the operating table.

The man to the left of the chief is smiling and nodding. It encourages me so I start to loosen up and talk mostly to him. The man to the right of the chief keeps a scowl on his face the whole time. When I'm done, the chief smiles warmly and thanks me heartily. In fact, everyone is thanking me. I kind of like that about the Liberians.

My escort then takes me to an empty office and asks me to write out my statement. I finish quickly, but then think I must have put the wrong date. Surely it can't have been the 22nd, it has to have been longer then that. I try to call Gillian to confirm but I can't get through. I just change my statement to the 15th. I later confirm it really was the 22nd. But for some reason in the moment, I'm uncertain and nervous.

I sit around for 15 minutes until my escort comes back to take min into the commission's room again. Everyone is laughing and joking about whether they'll be able to read my doctor's writing. I'm starting to feel really comfortable. The man assigned to read my statement does have some difficulty. Another man goes over to help. When they've finished, they open up the floor for questions such as the following:

"Have you ever removed a bullet form someone?"

"No."

"Was the colon touched?"

"Just the rectum which is the last part of the colon."

"You mention that the holes in the intestines were caused by a projectile such as a bullet, have you dealt with ballistics before?"

"Yes, I've treated gun shot wounds, just never taken a bullet out as it's not always necessary. Can I draw on the board?"

They agree and motion me up to the dry erase board. I trace out the digestive tract and point out why the injuries could only be caused by a bullet; how the bullet could pierce the skin, go through the small intestines and enter the rectum; and why the shape and size of the holes makes me confident it was a bullet as a knife or an arrow would leave a different type of wound.

Now the room feels really warm. All around people are nodding and saying "that's enough". "Thank you's" come from all around. I'm kind of embarrassed about how thankful they are, and yet it's nice too.

They call Dr. Sonii back in and we walk outside into the rain . The van picks us up and drives us back to the hospital. Titus is released that same day to go home,. He has recovered completely from his initial surgery and his colostomy is functioning normally. He'll have the colostomy take-down in 4-6 weeks.

If all goes well...

Deception
September 4

Once again I find myself ignoring my initial instinct and letting myself be convinced by a good story.

Phillip calls me outside. "Emergency in de car," he says.

I walk outside, pulling on gloves with a snap as I go. The woman is lying in the back seat of a beat up yellow taxi with a small crowd family members pushing in, all eager to tell me the "story." I glance in and see a critically ill, semi-conscious patient breathing heavily. A female relative holds her floppy head as it falls against the back seat.

I piece together the following story from the different people all trying to talk at once. She had malaria ten days ago which was treated with a three day course of Artemether/Lumafantrine, a common first-line therapy. Four days ago she had a miscarriage and bled heavily that evening. Yesterday, she went into the Benson Hospital where a doctor told them she needed an emergency D&C. The father paid the US$ 200 and the procedure was done. She stopped bleeding.

Today, however, her breathing became labored and she started to fade in and out of consciousness. The doctor told them she needed a blood transfusion and that their lab couldn't do it. He referred them to SDA Cooper Hospital.

In the back of my mind a still small voice is trying to whisper "where's the referral slip?" but that quickly gets suppressed by the good story I've just heard. How could they make all that up? I ask the typical screening questions about vomiting, fever, diarrhea, etc. They all adamantly shake their heads.

"No, she doesn't have any of that."

I motion for them to bring her in. She kind of stumbles up the steps, supported between two relatives. I have her wash her hands in chlorine water. I see her slump down as they now drag her through the door, past the benches in the waiting room and into the first exam room on the left.

They lay her on the exam table. She starts to seize and then stops breathing. The family starts to wail immediately. I roughly push them away shouting.

"Let me do my job, will you?"

I start doing CPR, half-heartedly I admit. I stop and check her pulse. The carotid artery is faintly pulsating. I keep pushing on her chest to force air in and out of her lungs. Not deep and rapid like compressions for the heart, but enough to get some air movement. I start calling for nursing help. R.B. And Vivian struggle to get an IV. I figure if we can just get some IV fluids in her and some blood maybe we can save her.

All along her arms are deep purple bruises. It wants to set off some alarm bells in my head, but I quickly silence them and keep up the resuscitation efforts. We pull the bed away from the table so the nurses can look for IVs on both arms. No success.

I have one of them take over chest compressions while I search for a femoral vein. I find it but have to hold it in a certain position or it stops. I get a dose of adrenaline in before the cannula moves and stops working. Her heart is beating stronger now. She's having some spontaneous, albeit weak, respiratory efforts.

I call for oxygen. At some point, Gillian shows up after finishing an appendectomy upstairs. The oxygen tank is missing the handle to open it. Otis runs to get another one. Habakuk, finally finds a small IV in her right hand and we start running in some fluids. Jeff has now arrived and is drawing blood to do a cross-match for a blood transfusion.

The nurses have changed shift so now it's Philip and Habakuk replacing R.B. and Vivian. I think the woman might still be bleeding from her miscarriage. I order some oxytocin to be given intramuscularly. We've finally got oxygen going and she's breathing on her own with a good pulse. Jeff has two bags of blood available. The first one is up and running and almost in.

"Bring in a family member," I ask a Philip.

Just as the sister walks in the door the patient seizes again and stops breathing.

"Get her out of here!" I point to the sister and we restart our efforts.

Finally, we succeed in getting her breathing and oxygenating well with a strong heartbeat and pulses. I call in the father. He is overjoyed and thanks us profusely. I'm happy. This is why we still do this CPR stuff, because sometimes it actually works. The second bag of blood is in, a recheck of her hemoglobin finds a stable 9 g/dl.

We've been working on her for two hours. The sister comes back in. We start talking. I ask some more questions. Suddenly, she starts talking about how she's had vomiting, watery diarrhea and fevers at home. I nervously look at the patients arms with the huge bruises. I notice all the places we tried to find IV access still oozing. I pick her her wrap and see that there's oozing from where we gave her the shot of Oxytocin.

I go ballistic, realizing she probably has Ebola. "What are you trying to do, get us all killed?" I scream. "Lies, all lies! Why didn't you tell us the truth."

The sister and father weakly try to give excuses: "We didn't know, I wasn't there..."

"The whole family was there when you were denying vomiting, diarrhea, and fever...don't lie! It won't help you or her! Take her out now!"

I'm sure she has Ebola! I'm starting to freak. I'm exhausted and feel like I've now put how many staff at risk? How could I ignore my instinct? If a staff member dies of Ebola, I'll feel responsible. I feel like for the first time I've had a serious exposure and my stomach is in knots. I rush home, take a shower and soak my scrubs in a red, hospital smelling disinfectant I find on a shelf in the shower.

The patient dies almost immediately on being carried out the hospital doors. The father comes back to the steel bars now keeping him out.

"Doctuh? Yo' di' yo' bes'. I come back tomorrow to settle accounts on our deposit."

I want to scream, "Is that all you can say after lying and exposing us all to a deadly plague!" But I keep my mouth shut and just stare.

Later that night, my sleep is troubled by fearful dreams. I wake up with my heart beating out of my chest. It's still dark outside. I kneel with my face to the floor and sob. I cry out to God for mercy, mostly for the staff, but that He will also spare my life from this plague.

James Appel, MD

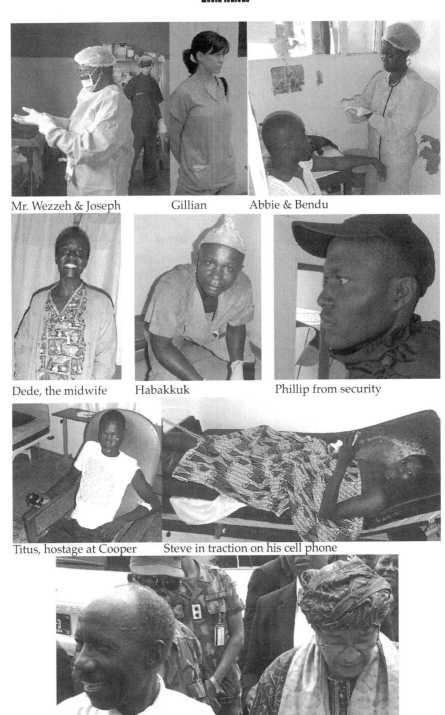

Mr. Wezzeh & Joseph   Gillian   Abbie & Bendu

Dede, the midwife   Habakkuk   Phillip from security

Titus, hostage at Cooper   Steve in traction on his cell phone

Mr. Wennie & President Ellen Johnson Sirleaf on her visit to SDA Cooper Hospital

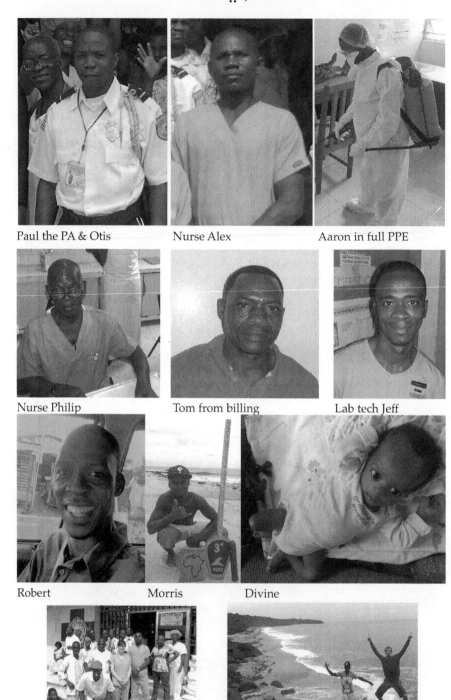

Stabbed

September 6

Yesterday, after the scare doing CPR on the probable Ebola patient, I turn away more people than I probably should have. It's amazing what fear of lies, Ebola and the unknown will do. After work last night, I settled in at home for some reflection. I tried to calm my spirit with music and reading, nothing worked. Then I finally just fell on my face. I sobbed and sobbed until my shot nerves were exhausted and calmed. Then I slept.

This morning, despite the vicious rain storm pounding the hospital, I see things clearer. My spirit is back on track and fear has been pushed to the side again.

Fortunately, there are only seventeen inpatients. I quickly go through rounds. Unfortunately, the boy I gave my rare B- type blood to three days ago passed in the night. His cerebral malaria just overwhelmed his internal organs and they all shut down.

The man with the liver abscess I put a drain in yesterday has had 400mL of thick pus come out. He's feeling a lot better.

Steve, the boy in traction for a femur fracture greets me with a big smile. Always before he's been crying, whining and begging for me to let him go home. His mom and grandma want to let a traditional healer have a go at it. I've been alternately stalling, cajoling and threatening the family members.

I've said that if Steve leaves against medical advice, I won't pull out the traction pin. Then I ask who will do it? That bought me a couple of days. Today, he is pain free and smiling saying he's willing to stay. I've also convinced him to stay by promising that the instruments and materials to do surgery are on their way. Adventist Health International is providing them in partnership with SIGN Fracture Care International.

I go home and relax. I listen to some talks and some music. I read some more in several of the books I've been reading. I take a little nap.

I get called back to the hospital in the early afternoon. A woman is out in the car. She is four months pregnant and they say she has "no blood." This sounds initially like some kind of sick deja vu from Thursday night. However, I go out to the taxi. This time the woman looks tired, but not sick. She has no evidence of bleeding from anywhere. Her conjunctiva are actual pale, as are her palms and soles.

She does have a fever.

I listen for any warning signs from my gut, instinct or still small voice. I hear only silence encouraging me to admit her. We get an IV going with a loading dose of Quinine. Two blood donors are available as well as an extra bag of O+ blood in the lab fridge.

Gillian and I then go out to a café to meet with Cameron, a veteran doc with MSF (Doctors Without Borders). He fills us in on what they're doing in the fight against Ebola. The grim reality is that Ebola is still on the upward side of the growth curve. He's with the Parisian section of MSF. Their role is to help the health care institutions, especially the hospitals like ours that are still open, to have better infectious control measures. He gives us a lot of good advice and promises to come with his team to the hospital in a week or so.

I go back just in time for Otis to call me about an emergency. A tall man is standing in front of the main entrance clutching a bloody shirt to his neck. His shorts are spattered with large patches of drying blood. His shorter brother is anxious and quickly states that he was stabbed in the neck about half an hour ago.

I bring him in, holding pressure myself over the neck with a gloved hand. Alex comes down from the inpatient ward and starts an IV. The young man appears to be hemodynamically stable. His lungs are clear. His conjunctiva are a normal color, meaning he probably hasn't lost too much blood.

Once the IV lines are in and fluids boluses running, I gently take away the shirt compressing the wound. A pool of dark blood wells up. I quickly put more pressure on with some gauze, directly over the wound. The bleeding instantly stops. I have Alex hold pressure while I go tell Gillian. t's her day off and she's with her "adopted" baby, Divine, that she watches every Saturday. She states we can explore it under local anesthesia.

I go back and we have the man walk upstairs. I've already got the theater ready. I turned on the lights, placed a drape on the operating table, unlocked the anesthesia cabinet, started the A/C and put on my hat and mask. Alex and I lay the man down. I pump up the bed until it's a comfortable height for me.

I get the local anesthetic ready in a 10cc syringe. I give the patient 10mg of IV Diazepam. Then, I take off the gauze. Having had about 10 minutes of direct pressure, the bleeding has stopped. Maybe it wasn't that serious after all. The wound looks shallow and wide, like a glancing blow.

I infiltrate the skin with the 10cc of Lidocaine and then prep it with Betadine. I'm too rough with my application of the Betadine as dark blood starts pouring out of the wound again. I quickly apply direct pressure again with one hand. I move on to anesthetize the small laceration on his lower sternum. I'd noticed it earlier. Since it was very superficial and barely bleeding, I'd ignored it until now.

I drape the neck and sternum with sterile towels, put on sterile gloves and then have Alex remove the gauze. The bleeding has stopped again. I raise the lower skin margin with forceps. I see a decent sized superficial vein running along the platysma muscle that was lacerated but is currently not bleeding. I do a figure of eight stitch around it to make sure it doesn't re-bleed. I close the platysma, subcutaneous tissues and skin with running sutures.

I explore the sternal wound and make sure it's not deep. I irrigate thoroughly and close with simple sutures. I'm about done when the man shows me his right thumb. It has a 2 cm knife wound on it that I suture as well.

I'm cleaning up when I notice crepitus under the skin over his left upper chest. Could the knife have gone down and punctured his left lung? I don't have x-ray. Instead, I have Alex bring me a stethoscope from the nurse's station. The patient's breath sounds are equal on both sides. Also, his O2 sats have remained 99% on room air the whole procedure. He's breathing easily. If it is a pneumothorax, it's small and asymptomatic. I elect not to put in a chest tube.

I then go to my office and Skype for over an hour with my family. I enjoy watching my kids run around, play and act silly.

The next morning, Sunday, I awake with a bit of a panic. What if the man got worse overnight and no one noticed? I get up, even though I'm exhausted and it's supposed to be my day off. I go up to the hospital. The man is lying comfortably in the bed. He's breathing normally. His lungs still sound symmetric and clear. I breath a sigh of relief and go home, ready for my day off.

Body
September 8

It scared the kitchen staff when they first realized what it was.

Dr. Martin admitted the man with vomiting, fever and a diagnosis of presumed malaria and hepatitis. Once admitted, he started vomiting up blood. I informed the family that he'd have to be taken to the Ebola center for testing. The staff put on protective gear and took him out to the side courtyard in a wheelchair. The brother of the patient went to find a vehicle. Within a few minutes of getting outside, the man died.

Dr. Sonii called the Ministry of Health Ebola hotline. They promised to send out a vehicle that same day or the next day at the latest. We covered the body with a surgical drape and leave him in the wheelchair. No one showed up.

The next morning the kitchen staff prepared breakfast. While cleaning up, they suddenly noticed there's a body under the drape. They fled in panic. The inpatients were left without food for the rest of the day. Dr. Sonii called the Ebola hotline all afternoon, still no one came.

It had rained all day and night on the body sitting outside. The staff were starting to get worried. Sunday comes, two days after the man's death. The body is still there. It's my day off, but Gillian comes at around 8:00AM to say that none of the staff have come in to work. I get up and go out to help her. By about 9:00AM, most of the staff have arrived. I look out the window of my office. I see that the body is still there, mostly covered with the drape. Just the ashen, stiff feet are sticking out from under it.

Mr. Wennie, the business manager pokes his head in. "What we gonna do about de body?"

"I think someone needs to go in person to the Ebola Crisis center and refuse to leave until someone comes to take the body."

"Yeah, it's a good idea. I will do it." And Mr. Wennie heads off.

Ebola-iculous

Since I have the day off, I go home and sleep till noon. I spend the afternoon at the beach. That evening I have a wonderful pizza dinner with an old mentor, friend and colleague from Ventura County Medical Center. John Fankhauser, MD is now the administrator of the ELWA Hospital. He has helped spearhead the efforts to treat Ebola patients. They have their own Ebola Treatment Unit (ETU) with about 40 beds and 70 patients. MSF is now setting up a 160 bed ETU on the ELWA campus.

John also was the one who personally treated Dr. Kent Brantley before he was evacuated to Emory University. There, Kent made a complete recovery from his own encounter with Ebola. Needless to say, we had some very interesting conversations.

I go back to work the next day and the body is finally gone.

Later that morning, Titus comes back. It seems he's forgot we spent four hours operating on him to save his life after a gun shot wound to the abdomen. He had recovered fully and was sent home after nine days in the hospital.

He is back for his one week, post-discharge check up. He's been busy during that one week. Titus has become a media sensation in a country who's TV and Radio can't wait to bash the government. A staff member here at Cooper Hospital saw the TV interview where Titus explained that Cooper Hospital had done nothing for him. For dramatic effect he then lifted up his shirt to reveal the colostomy and its bag filled with stool. Everyone ooooohhhh'd and aaaaahhhh'd at the obvious evidence of our incompetence.

Titus went on to deceive the public by stating that we had kicked him out of the hospital. He said it was because the government had refused to pay his medical bills. Therefore he needed to be evacuated to the USA or Europe for proper medical care.

The media never bothered to check out the other side of the story, namely ours. Of course, his bill was paid. We don't let patients leave the hospital unless their bills are paid otherwise we'll never get reimbursed. Secondly, he would've received no better care anywhere else in the world. We had told him that the colostomy was a necessary, temporary measure to divert his stool so the wound in his rectum could heal. But to an uneducated and ignorant public I can see what they would think seeing stool coming out the side of someone's belly!

So, Titus is back for his checkup, accompanied by the commissioner of West Point. I tell him that he can live for many years with a colostomy. There is no hurry to take it down. Therefore, until he apologizes publicly and gives credit to Cooper Hospital for saving his life, we won't see him.

Titus gets sullen and whiny. He starts threatening to go kill himself. He gets up and goes across the street to catch a motorcycle taxi demonstrating his obviously good physical condition. His brother chases after him trying to scream some reason into his childish, spoiled brain.

I go back in the hospital. I have a meeting with John at ELWA to meet their surgeon. I get in Gillian's Honda CRV and take off.

When I get back, Gillian informs me that the government is requesting that we hospitalize Titus until we do the colostomy take down. This will help allay concerns that the government is not taking care of him medically. The hospitalization will also serve to keep him away from the media.

As much as I don't want to be seeing that young man every day for the rest of the month, I do admit it's a good plan. When his colostomy is put back in and he's fully healed, we can call the media on his release date, tell our side of the story and show him 100% better.

Titus is back. This time around, no general ward for him. He sits resignedly in a private room, watching TV, and waiting...

Pregnancy
September 8-9

    I'm called out to see a pregnant woman. This is her fourth pregnancy. She states she's at "10 months". She's been leaking vaginal fluid for 3 days. She also has fever and uterine contractions. She denies vomiting, diarrhea or other suspicious symptoms of Ebola (unless she's lying). I admit her to labor and delivery. Her cervix is only dilated 4 cm according to Dede, the midwife. I put her on antibiotics, a Quinine drip and do an ultrasound. I find twins with an estimated gestational age of 34 weeks! The first is vertex and the second is breech. Both are very much alive.

    As I'm walking out of labor and delivery, I poke my head into the postpartum room. Sarah, the woman I'd admitted two days ago is lying in her hospital bed. We transfused her four units of blood. She is doing better but still complaining of abdominal pain. I hadn't been able to find a fetal heart beat on admission. I wasn't surprised since she had a hemoglobin of 3 and malaria.

    Because of the early age of her pregnancy, I didn't feel an ultrasound was urgent the night of admission. I figured she would probably miscarry shortly. If not, I'd planned to scan her the next day. Unfortunately, I wasn't thinking that the next day was my day off. I'd completely forgotten about it until now.

    "Have you miscarried yet?" I ask.

    Sarah shakes her head. I go get the ultrasound to see if by some miracle the fetus is still alive or if we need to help the miscarriage happen.

    I place the ultrasound on her slightly swollen lower abdomen and find a mass. The fetus is dead. Suddenly, I realize that this mass is not in the uterus. It's an ectopic pregnancy! I can now easily find the empty uterus. There's lots of free fluid in the abdomen which is most certainly blood. I call in the OR team: Mr. Wezzeh, Joseph and News, the anesthetist on call.

I inform Gillian. She wants to do the case so I just help get Sarah ready. The midwives get busy finding IVs, putting up fluids and inserting a foley catheter. Meanwhile, Gillian and I get some blood bags and drain the blood from her abdomen in preparation for an auto transfusion. We get one and a half units. Once the team arrives, we wheel Sarah's off to surgery.

I go down to my office and Skype with my wife, also named Sarah. Jeff, the lab tech who wants to study medicine, comes down from the operating theater fully suited up in protective gear.

"Dr. Seton want to see yo'," he says.

I hurry upstairs, putting on my mask and surgical cap as I go. It turns out Gillian's already removed the dead fetus and remnants of the placenta. She just has a couple of minor questions. I confirm her ideas and watch a bit before going back out.

Just outside the theater is the labor and delivery room. I stop in to see how the pregnant mom with twins is doing.

"You want boys or girls?" I ask her.

She smiles shyly and says "Girls.

There is no cervical change in the last four hours. I start an oxytocin drip and go back down stairs. I wave to Joseph and Mr. Wezzeh as they leave. After a few more minutes I go up to check on the labor patient.

As I glance over the chart I note that Dede has ordered lab tests including an HIV test which is positive. Neither Jeff nor Dede had mentioned it to me. Maybe Dede didn't even notice since they use code here: Comb's test positive = HIV positive.

We immediately start the national protocol for prevention of transmission of HIV from the mother to the fetus. I also stop the Oxytocin drip. I call up Joseph and Mr. Wezzeh. I ask them to come in at 6:00AM tomorrow for the c-section. Since the babies appear to be doing well, I want to get in a few more doses of the antiretrovirals to protect them from HIV before delivery.

The next morning, I'm awake at 5:15AM. I get up, eat cold oatmeal and go up to prepare for the c-section. We finally are ready at 7:30AM but the anesthetist is still not here.

"He not gonna be heuh on tahme," Mr. Wezzeh tells me. "We shouldna wait..."

I sit the patient up on the operating table, prep her back with Betadine and put on sterile gloves. I draw up the spinal anesthetic, find the interspace I'm looking for and insert the spinal needle. I go a bit too far and get blood back when I withdraw the stylet. I move the needle out a couple millimeters and get clear spinal fluid. I inject the anesthetic and have her lie down.

Ebola-iculous

I monitor her for about 20 minutes. Her blood pressure drops slightly. I open up the IV fluids in her two 18G cannulas. Her pressure comes back up quickly. Then her heart beat starts to slow down to the 50s. Then it briefly goes into the 40s. I draw up some adrenaline and have it on the ready. However, she is conscious, talking and has a normal oxygen saturation and blood pressure. After a few minutes the heart beat goes back up to over 60 per minute. I feel reassured and go scrub up for surgery.

During the whole case I keep my ear tuned to the sound of the pulse oximeter. My eye keeps glancing at the heart rate and blood pressure. I make a quick midline incision down to and through the fascia. With my fingers I stretch and tear my way through the peritoneum. I'm quickly into the abdominal cavity looking down on the shining uterus.

I enlarge the incision inferiorly with scissors, making sure to spare the bladder. I dissect out a bladder flap. Mr. Wezzeh protects the bladder with a retractor while I open up the uterus. Amniotic fluid bursts into the surgical field.

She hasn't had rupture of membranes after all! That's good news for the twins! They will be much less likely to get HIV from their mom if the membranes have been intact this whole time. I pull out a full term girl who is flexing and soon screaming in fury at being brought into the world.

I open up the second amniotic sac. The second girl is breech. I extract her feet and legs. Keeping traction on the feet, I sweep out one arm at a time. I put my finger in the tiny mouth and pull out her head. She's much smaller than her twin, yet also curls up with good muscle tone.

Dede has to work to get the second one to cry, but she eventually does. Meanwhile, I've sutured the uterus closed. I ask the mother if she wants more children and she says "No." I willingly tie her tubes. I close the fascia and skin. Mr. Wezzeh puts on a dressing while I go home to eat second breakfast.

Blur

September 11

I'm losing track of time. Cases and patients are coming in and out of my memory. I can't even remember sequences of events or what day it all came to pass. I'm not sure now if things happened in a day or a week or what. It's all becoming a blur of images flashing through my mind as I try and grab some food here and some sleep there (and the occasional surf thrown in for good measure.)

A tiny 16 year old is referred from an outside clinic after three days of labor. The cervix is completely dilated and the baby's head very molded. There are no fetal heart tones. I set up for a symphysiotomy. I inject the skin and subcutaneous tissues down to the cartilage of the pubis. I slice down, cut through the cartilage and have my assistants put gentle downward pressure on the legs until the pelvis splits apart a few centimeters.

The baby is still having a difficult time coming out. I add oxytocin to the saline drip. I inject the labia and do a mediolateral episiotomy. By the time the huge, dead baby comes out, the mother also has a massive periurethral tear all the way up into the symphysiotomy wound.

I start to repair the wounds. I'm leaning over from the side with almost no light. Mr. Wezzeh has Gillian's headlamp which helps tremendously, as long as he's looking where I'm working. I begin the repair with the sympysiotomy wound which I easily close in two layers.

I begin work on the periurethral tear. The anatomy is distorted and she's bleeding heavily. I hold pressure and ask Mr. Wezzeh to bring some more lap sponges. I massage the uterus and ask Dede to give more oxytocin and ergometrine. Finally, the bleeding slows down.

I finally am able to pull the urethra back to the side wall and then close the vaginal mucosa. The repair of the episiotomy is easy after that. I run the suture from inside to out and back again in a continuous line.

The patient looks pale afterwards. Jeff is there since it's early evening already. He does a hemoglobin. It's 3 g/dl. She needs blood. The family has gone home. Jeff knows someone who is willing to donate blood for a price. He comes in and gives. Seems kind of sketchy to me since we can't test for Ebola. But it's an emergency. The worst thing is the bag isn't even completely full.

We need more blood. The sister refuses to donate. Everyone else is "far away" and of course there's the curfew because of Ebola. I put her on a quinine drip and hope she makes it through the night. Did I mention she came in with fever? I'm glad her malaria smear is positive. I'd hate to think she had Ebola with all that blood flying around.

* * * * *

The outpatient department is crowded. I'm called out to see three guys from the same neighborhood who've all started vomiting since arrival at the hospital. We've built a crude lean-to against the outside wall of the hospital with a tarp stretched over the top to shield the patients from the sun or rain. They have to wait outside often for hours waiting to be screened and seen by a provider.

No one seems to be too concerned about the vomiting. People are still sitting in relatively close proximity to the three men. I take the first guy's temperature: 39.1 C. He looks Ebola-ish with red eyes, a haunting stare and sunken cheek bones. Even though he denies diarrhea I don't believe him. I refer all three to the ELWA Ebola Treatment Unit.

* * * * *

I'm called out to see a woman in a black pickup truck. She looks like death warmed over. She's unconscious and has labored breathing. Her conjunctiva look normal and she has no gingival bleeding. The family of course denies nausea and vomiting. They say she just "fell off" last night (meaning she passed out). I check her temperature: 41.3 C!

I'm still amazed at my continuing gullibility as I have them bring her in to the ER. After all it's probably malaria right? I personally start an IV on each arm. I put up Dextrose in one line and Saline in the other. I then start a Quinine drip and have R.B. give IV Ceftriaxone. I go away.

I'm at lunch when R.B. calls. "De woman throwin' out," she says.

I go in and she's doing slightly better...except for still being unconscious and now lying in her own vomit. I want to send her away immediately, but the R.B. speaks up.

"We stahted de drip. Le's do labs an' see wha' she got."

I call in Jeff who draws some blood in full protective gear. A few minutes later he brings back the results: negative. The black truck that brought her has left. I have the caretaker call them back. I go see some other patients.

Otis calls me when the truck arrives. I explain to the family leader that I suspect Ebola. He says he's part of the Ebola Task Force and pulls out an infrared thermometer from his pocket. He informs me he checks everyone's temperature all the time. He assures me she didn't have a fever before. He agrees to take her to ELWA. I prepare a referral form. I get protective kits for the two people who will carry her out.

I go and clear the lobby by having everyone sit over in the corner. I go outside and move the waiting patients all under the overhang. One young man is angry.

"Who dis whahte man? Tink he can talk lahke dat. He can jus' ohduh me aroun'?"

Patience not being my virtue, I don't bridle my tongue. I quickly find myself in a useless wars of words. I also have the other cars move away from the black truck. When the coast is clear I have the team bring out the woman.

When the fully protected Ebola task force man sees that I've had everyone move aside he is angry and shouts at me.

"Ya makin' sometin' outta nottin'! Makin' everyone tink she got Ebola o' sometin! It not rahte!"

I can't help but yell back: "This is why Ebola is running havoc in this country! When even people on the task force can't admit that someone is suspicious and take precautionary measures!"

He'd have preferred to take her out without gear and through the thick of a crowd to avoid suspicion!

* * * * *

A baby comes in after midnight with stridor. The tiny five month old chest is flailing in and out with severe substernal retractions. There is no air movement in the lung fields. I diagnose croup. I inject dexamethasone in her thigh and start an adrenaline nebulizer treatment. I have to give continuous treatments for over an hour, holding the mask myself over the tiny mouth and nose before air starts moving past the swollen trachea and into the lungs. The baby is very chubby and the mom assures me that she's breastfed exclusively. I'm not surprised. I order frequent nebulizer treatments and leave her in the hands of Philip, the nurse on duty.

*****

I'm at home. I hear a pounding on the door. It's a nurse's aide.

"Doc, come to OB! A woman got twins! De fuhst one breech an' half way out an' stuck!"

I pull on scrubs and run up and down the maze of stairs to Labor and Delivery. I put on gloves quickly, grab the baby's tiny feet and pull with all my strength. The body inches out until I can hook my index finger over the anterior arm and swing it out. I give the baby a quick twist so the posterior, undelivered arm comes anterior and deliver that with some serious straining.

I put a finger in the baby's mouth, tilt the chin down and pull even harder and the baby comes out with a pop! He's floppy and I'm afraid it's too late. I instinctively start chest compression. The on call midwife is vigorously rubbing and drying the newborn.

The baby takes a gasp. I keep going with CPR.

"Get me an ambu bag...quick!"

Before the midwife can get it, the baby is taking small breaths. I continue to suction the nose and throat, stimulate vigorously and pound furiously on the tiny chest. The skin pinks up. The legs and arms start to contract and the boy lets out a lusty yell!

I turn to the mom and notice she still looks very pregnant. We're not done! There's twins! I rupture the membranes and feel that it's a vertex presentation. The midwife should be ok with this one. I go back home and eat breakfast. That's right, it was early in the morning. Like I said, it's all running together in a blur.

Liberianese
September 12

"Dere's a puhsun in de cah," says Habakuk at my office door.

"I'm coming." I put on my gloves and walk down the dimly lit hallway to the dark waiting area.

Outside the metal bars securing the entrance to the hospital is a brand new Land Cruiser with about ten people inside and out.

"What's going on," I ask as I approach and see a 60 year old man sitting in the back seat. He has an obvious left sided facial droop and his left arm hangs limply in his lap.

"Preshuh," says the fat woman sitting next to him on his left.

"Is that all? What else?"

The family members give each other quick sidelong glances as if to say "Wha' de white man sayin?"

"He feelin' weeeeaak," finally suggests someone hopefully.

"I can see that. Everyone who comes to the hospital is weak. And I'm sure he has high blood pressure, but what brought him in specifically tonight?"

I see the light bulb go on for the young man looking over the head rest into the back from the passenger seat. "He fell off!"

"When?" I ask having learned enough Liberianese to know he meant the man fell down.

"Las' night," pipes up a young girl who's come into the back of the Land Cruiser to get a better view of the entertaining spectacle of trying to understand the pale foreigner.

I switch to my best Liberianese: "His skin can be hot?"

The fat lady shakes her head vigorously waving her right index finger back and forth as she tut-tuts in her throat. "No, his skin canna be hot."

"His stomach running? He can throw out?" Everyone joins in the denial of diarrhea and vomiting.

Ebola-iculous

"His head can hurt? He can toilet? He can pee pee?" This time there's nods all around. I hear positive affirmations coming from all directions to my questions about headache, defecation and urination.

"Yeah, his head can HUHT!"

"He toilet free!"

"He can pee pee fast fast!"

I explain that he's had a stroke a there's not much we can do. The only things we can offer are to help him control his blood pressure, give him aspirin and have him change his diet to a whole food plant based regime. I give them a prescription and go back inside. I walk upstairs to do evening rounds on the inpatient service.

I poke my head in to the post c-section room. "How are things?"

"I'm trying," speaks up the woman who had a seizure last night, probably from malaria or late manifestation of eclampsia.

I finish rounds and go home. I've only been tossing and turning for a few hours when Habakuk is back. It's 2:00AM.

"Dere so' woma' in de cah."

I go to see the next emergency. Theres' a woman almost as wide as she is tall waddling up to the front steps. With one hand she hold her lower back. The other hand rests on top of an obviously full term pregnancy. She announces her presence loudly as she approaches.

"Oh, Lawd hehhhhp me! I been in labuh fo' fahhhhve dayz! De mi'wife say I shouldna go to de hospital 'cause mah livuh buhhhhnin' up. But I say I canna stay in huh house one mo' nahhhhht! I goin' to de hospital... but ma hospital close'. So I come to de Cooooooopuh Hospital. Mah skin not hot, I not throwin' out, mah stomach not runnin'."

I hate to interrupt her, but I need to ask her a few questions, "Is this your first pregnancy?"

"No, Lawwwwd no! I got one 18 yeuh ol' dattuh a' home. Dis de secon' one. Dat mi'wife she give me some tablet insahhhhde to make de baby come. Den she give me some injehhhhkshun but it not workin' I tell huh I gohhhhhin' to Coooooopuh."

"Follow me."

We go upstairs. She waddles after me moaning and groaning the whole way. It's right before midnight. First, I do an ultrasound and confirm the baby is alive. Then I spend a couple hours adjusting an Oxytocin drip to try and get her contractions going. She should be able to deliver vaginally. She is 8 cm dilated on arrival.

Finally, I get everything arranged and it appears she is progressing. I leave at about 4:00AM. As I walk back home I have a nagging doubt deep down that I should've just done a c-section and been done with it. Then I'd know the baby would be alright. If she's waited 18 years for her second child and is now 36 years old herself, this is probably her last chance to have another child. But I'm exhausted and I go home and fall asleep.

At 7:00AM I wake up. I don't want to get up, but I feel compelled to go check on the woman. She's probably delivered by now since no one has come to get me. But it will ease my mind to check.

I pull on my scrubs groggily. I walk painfully up the three flights of steps to the inpatient ward and then down the half flight to the labor and delivery. The woman is still on the table.

"Mohnin' Doc! You got to do anudduh ultrasoun'," announces one of the midwives. "We can' fin' de fetal hahht tones."

If I wasn't so exhausted my heart would probably sink to my shoes, but I feel indifferent and resigned. I pull out the ultrasound and start looking. It's difficult to see with the woman's copious abdominal girth. I can't seem to find any heart tones. Then, deep on the screen, I see something. I move the probe around a little and definitely find a fetal heart beating normally!

"She got Caput!" announces the other midwife. I do a vaginal exam and find the head still very high up. The fetal head is very deformed, trying to cram through a tiny pelvis. I get all the gear together and perform my fourth symphysiotomy since arriving here over a month ago.

Within 15 minutes after the procedure, the woman has delivered a floppy baby covered in thick pea-soup colored meconium. I aspirate the mouth and nose with a bulb suction. Still no breathing. I start chest compressions as I wipe up all the gunk from the baby's gray skin.

I'm just going through the motions as instinct kicks in. I've got no adrenaline left. The last few days has depleted my reserves. I don't even have the strength to yell at the midwives to bring the ambu bag and oxygen quickly.

Miraculously, the baby finally starts gasping a little and gets slightly less gray. The midwife confirms a slow heartbeat with a stethoscope. I keep up the chest compressions. Now the heartbeat is faster and the newborn girl is taking shallow breaths. We take her into the OR to give her oxygen and she pinks up.

Finally, she cries after a lot of stimulation. Her muscle tone is improving as well. I go back to Labor and Deliver to remove the placenta. I suture up the wound and go back home. I'm just in time to cook and eat some French Toast before getting called for another "puhsun in de cah."

Conjunctiva
September 13

I'm glad to see the nurses in the Emergency Room are wearing full protective gear. R.B. is just putting a rubber glove around the forearm of the four year old boy, getting ready to start an IV line. The bottle of IV fluids is hanging on a rusted IV pole that no longer extends. The fluid inside is yellow. The nurses have a habit of putting Vitamin B-Complex into the Quinine drips to help identify them. That way it is less likely for someone to accidentally turn up the rate as giving Quinine too quickly can be lethal.

"Stop!" I warn. "The malaria smear was negative. Let's just give him the shot of Ceftriaxone. I'll write a prescription for some tablets and we can send him home."

Three pairs of eyes look back at me under caps and over masks, acknowledging that they've understood my unspoken fear: the child now has a high suspicion of having Ebola. If it's not malaria causing the fever, headaches and lethargy, then in Monvrovia in 2014 Ebola goes to the top of the list. Adding to the suspicion is the fact that his conjunctiva are too red for malaria which usually causes anemia and pallor.

I'm called out to see an "Emuhguhncy" in a car. It's a beat up red station wagon. A sophisticated, well-dressed man with short, white hair greets me.

"Good aftuhnoon doctuh, how de body?"

"Fine, how are you? What's happening with the girl?" I ask.

I peer into the back seat and see a 10 year old with a home knitted stocking cap pulled low over her forehead. She is conscious but is obviously not feeling well. She looks a little pale from here and her face is somewhat swollen.

A large woman from behind the distinguished gentlemen pipes up, probably the mother. "She sick fo' fo' day now. Her skin can be hahhht. A' naht she can feel cohhhhhld!" And she demonstrates by pulling her arms up in a shivering motion.

"...And she weeeeak. She got no appuhtite," adds another woman of unknown relation to the patient.

"Can she toilet normal?" I inquire. "Can she vomit, throw out?"

"No she not trowin' ou', but she toilet fast fast dis mohnin'."

"How many times she toilet?"

"Fo' tahms...she anemic."

I feel I've gotten a good history, surprisingly enough. I go to the other side of the station wagon and open the rear door. With a gloved finger, I examine what to me has become the most important part of the body diagnostically in this age of Ebola: the conjunctiva.

Sure enough, this girl's are redder then normal, especially considering I thought she might have malaria by the history. Of course, the four episodes of diarrhea this morning is atypical for malaria, but very typical for Ebola entering the later stages.

check her temporal temperature with the infrared thermometer "gun": 40.2 C. Not good. I feel a rush of sadness. I've turned away many suspected Ebola patients, but most of them are adults, somehow that makes it easier. But this one is a kid. What if it really is malaria, a treatable disease? Then I'm almost surely sending her to her death. But if it is Ebola she will most likely die regardless. And if she infects someone in the hospital, our whole operation will shut down and we won't be able to help anyone.

"You need to take her to MSF at ELWA Hospital. She needs to be tested for Ebola. I'll write a referral that will help you get in."

The family seems to have suspected that all along as they nod their heads in resignation. After writing the referral I come back out and the distinguished gentleman walks up to me.

"It too late today, they won' tes' huh 'til tomorrow. Dere pills you can gi' her tonaht?"

Sounds like a good idea, especially if it's malaria. I go back in, write a prescription and take it to the pharmacy to calculate the amount. I go back to the door and tell the man the amount:

"520 Liberian dollars for the tablets."

He goes back to the car and soon comes back with six 100 dollar bills. I take the money into billing, get his receipt and take it to the pharmacist. She should have gone home already but has asked the staff bus to wait so she can get this girl her meds. I hand them out to the white haired man and he drives off with the little girl.

Vivian asks me to come up to the wards. Apparently, a patient just admitted got word that a close friend just died of Ebola. This patient was admitted by Dr. Martin for esophagitis and was fortunately put in a private room. When I look at the chart I see Gillian's note which mentions "very red conjunctiva."

I go down the hall to N wing and open the door to N3. There on the floor lies a woman sprawled out, face down with a puddle of blood near her right arm. A steady drip is coming out from where her IV cannula used to be in her forearm. The IV tubing hangs pathetically from the IV pole, it's heavily taped and bloodied end limp against the tile.

"Hey! What's happening?"

The woman lifts up her head, groans and pulls herself to a sitting position on the floor.

"Can you talk? What's going on?" I repeat.

More animal like grunts come from her throat.as she lifts her eyes to look at me. I see what I dread most: bleary, injected, hyperemic, red conjunctiva. The woman won't speak. I start to yell:

"Ma'am, this isn't helping. You haven't died and we would like to help you. But we can't when you just throw yourself around!"

"I jus' wanna dahh now, dahh now…" moans the woman with more grunts and groans.

I go downstairs with the chart to see Dr. Martin in his air conditioned office. He sits behind a large wooden desk piled high with papers, talking on a fat smart phone.

"Yeah, heh de doctuh now," Dr. Martin looks over at me. "Dis de husband o' dat woman."

I pick up the phone and explain that his wife has gone psycho on us since hearing about a friend dying of Ebola and that her caretaker has abandoned her.

"You need to send someone to get her and take her to ELWA to get tested for Ebola…" I finish.

The man starts talking about an ambulance or something so I pass the phone back to Dr. Martin. Dr. Martin nods a bit and then makes sure the man understands what I said and that he should get an ambulance or something to pick up his wife.

"Dese people ah tricky. Dis man been mah mechanic fo' six yeauhs. She didn't soun' like Ebola at all. She ha' oral trush and I just put huh in fo' some IV hydrashun."

Later on, Gillian finds the woman slithering down the hall on her belly. Gillian calls and pays for an ambulance herself since the husband and other family haven't shown up. They've abandoned her.

Meanwhile, I'm called to see another patient who has been having fever and vomiting off and on for 4 days. They swear that "huh stomach no' running". When I finish the history, I turn to examine the patient lying face up on the back seat.

Ebola-iculous

I notice her lips are blue. I pull back her eyelids to look at her conjunctiva and they aren't red. But then again her pupils are fixed and dilated. She has no pulse and isn't breathing.

My first reaction is one of relief, I don't have to make a hard decision on whether to turn this patient away or not. She's dead on arrival. The family then opens up and tells the full story. It seems they were suspicious of Ebola all along and they want to take the body to be tested. I think it's a good move so I give them some advice.

"When you go to MSF at ELWA Hospital, tell them she had vomiting 5 times a day, diarrhea 10 times daily and a really high fever. Then they'll be sure to test her for Ebola. If you just tell them what you told me they may or may not do the test."

"You gettin' de white man?" asks a younger man to the others. "We got to tell dem she throwing out and huh stomach runnin' fast fast so dey will test huh. Tank you vehhy much, Doc."

And they drive off.

Shoulder

September 14

I'm sitting at home writing email when I hear the phone ring. I go into the kitchen and pick it up.

"Hello?"

"Yeah dey ga' pwobluhm inna laybuh roo'."

"Huh?" I demand.

"Laybuh, laybuh, complicashun…"

"Ok, ok I'm coming."

I go to the bedroom, rip off my shorts and t-shirt and pull on my scrubs. I grab my keys, slip on my crocs and lock the door behind me. Around the small courtyard, past Gillian's Honda CRV, through the narrow passage between the stairs and the basement wall, into the dark hallway leading to the kitchen, turn a 180 degree left and up two split level flights of stairs, then to the right in the main ward hallway, another quick right, under the curtains, down a half flight of steps next to a steep ramp, past the postpartum rooms and into labor and delivery. Upon entering the room, I see four gowned, booted, gloved, masked and hatted nurses, midwives and aides crowding around a large woman on the delivery table.

There is much screaming as Dede is pulling desperately on a large fetal head stuck outside the vulva. Another midwife is standing on a step stool putting all her weight into pushing on the uterus.

I understand instantly what's happened as I rush to put on gloves: shoulder dystocia. The anterior shoulder of the fetus is stuck behind the pubic bone of the mother's pelvis. Either the baby's too big or the mother's too small. I don't have time to put on full protective gear. I know I'm taking a risk here in the Ebola Capital of the World, but there's no time to waste.

I rush in and grab the head between my two palms. I try to pull downward as I shout at the midwife on the step stool:

"Push down on the pubic bone instead of the uterus!!!"

There is no room to pull down as the woman is in the middle of the delivery bed.

"Pull her down quickly to the end of the bed!"

There is pandemonium and not much happens. I grab under the woman's massive thighs and heave. Up and down I go slowly nudging the mass of flesh down the table. The others finally get the idea and pitch in until we get her butt to the edge of the table.

"Not like that!" I shout, noticing that the midwife only has a few fingers on the pubis and is barely pushing with bent elbows.

"You.." I point to John, a nurse's aide and the only other man in the room. "Get up here and push hard straight down…"

I immediately grab the head again and pull steadily but sturdily downward. The skin on the baby's face feels as cold as a piece of meat pulled from the fridge. Finally, there is some movement and the shoulder slowly pulls free. I then lift up to release the posterior shoulder and the baby slides out.

Immediately, there is an explosion of meconium, blood clots and amniotic fluid. I jump back but not quick enough. Some of the goulash splashes on my left thigh and all over my feet inside my crocs.

I place the newborn on the mother's abdomen and immediately begin chest compressions. One midwife is clamping and cutting the cord while the other grabs the ambu bag. When the baby is freed from the placenta, I lug the floppy mess over to the resuscitation table and continue CPR.

"Get me some oxygen!" I yell as someone goes to the Operating Theater to bring the large O2 tank there.

I keep up the CPR and call for a stethoscope which a nurse places in my ears. I stop CPR and listen to the small chest. I hear a faint heartbeat at about 80 beats per minute. I keep up CPR while Dede gives breaths with the ambu bag.

"Get some D50 into de rectum!" Dede orders.

"Great idea!" I confirm as I keep up chest compressions on the limp but pinking up chubby newborn.

I listen again and hear a fast heart beat. I stop CPR and take over giving breaths with the ambu bag. Oxygen arrives. John hooks it up to the ambu bag. I'm leaning over and my back is killing me. I want to keep listening to the baby's heart and respirations. Either I'm too tall, the table is too low or the stethoscope is too short.

"Get me some chlorine water and dump it over my feet, please!"

I soon get a soak on my feet and slosh around in the chlorine water in my crocs.

"Pour some on that junk on my leg too!"

And my thigh joins the wet chlorine party.

"Oh and some on my arm too!"

I notice some blood drops on my left arm which the nurse scrubs away. I never thought I'd have such an affection for chlorine! But here in Ebola Land, I really love the stuff.

The baby is cold and the incubator takes forever to heat up. We need to heat her up so we move the baby girl to her mother's belly and cover her up with blankets. She's breathing on her own now and pink, but still limp and not crying.

I go home, strip down and wash my scrubs by hand in an antiseptic solution. Then I take a cold shower, pouring water over my hunched over body with a metal cup dipped in a bucket. I stand up and let the water drip off my shoulders.

Stupid
September 15

"That is the stupidest thing I've ever seen! When are you going to learn? Did that really help you? Think about it, did you make things better? If not, try doing something different next time! Otherwise you're just being stupid! How old are you? Eighteen? Then start acting like an adult and not like a child!"

The young man is lying on the floor in the hallway of the hospital wards. His left leg is shorter than his right and deformed at the distal thigh. He has a metal pin sticking out both sides of the proximal end of his anterior tibia. He is bawling and whining like a child, blubbering on and on in barely comprehensible baby talk about wanting to go home and call his mommy.

In case you hadn't guessed, it's Steve.

He came in a few weeks ago with the femur fracture and wanted to have traditional healing done. We'd convinced him to stay in traction, telling him that the instruments would be coming shortly from SIGN Fracture Care International so we can do an operation to internally fix his broken bone.

Unfortunately, there's been delays in the shipment. Fortunately, after one week of pain and whining, Steve has been smiling and happy. His pain had been gone. And now I find him on the floor outside his room.

Steve, the charge nurse, tells me the story. Young Steve ripped off the rope attached to the pin that was keeping his leg out to length and tried to get up and stand. Since he'd been feeling so good, he thought he should be able to walk already.

In fact, yesterday he asked me if when he can start walking on his leg since it isn't hurting him anymore. I'd explained to him that it would be another month at least. He obviously knew better than the quack "whahte" doctor. He took things into his own hands.

After falling down, as could be expected without full bone

healing, he then began screaming, whining and begging to go home. To top it off, he then dragged himself out into the hallway before being stopped by the excruciating pain.

He's still blubbering and reaching for his phone. I take it out of his hand which produces a long howl with interspersed cries and whimpers from our spoiled boy. I go get some gloves and hand them out. Steve, Habakuk and I get him back into bed and hook him up to traction again despite his cursing and blithering. I arrange the leg back out to length and get it lined up in an anatomic position. I go to the nurses station and prescribe some pain killers. I hand baby Steve's phone to nurse Steve.

"Give this back to him when he's calmed down with the meds."

I go downstairs and a few minutes later am accosted in the lobby by Steve's brother. "Listen I need to talk to you…"

I'm in the middle of seeing an obstetrical emergency and I'm still peeved by Steve's behavior. My reply is rather brusque:

"I don't have time to talk to you about your stupid brother right now, I'm with another patient."

I guess I probably shouldn't have called Steve stupid, even if it was the truth. The brother gets very angry and starts yelling at me. I yell back a little. Tthe people in the lobby back me up and tell the man to wait outside. That is exactly what I've been trying to get him to do.

Once again, little Steve has stayed to get appropriate treatment for his fracture. But it's tough holding a spoiled brat against his will, even if it is for his own stupid good.

Clues

September 16

It starts to get crazy in the afternoon. I'm in Labor and Delivery adjusting an oxytocin drip on a woman in her first pregnancy. A local ante-natal clinic referred to us because she has a "big baby." Mr. Wezzeh and Joseph have just taken a woman with twins—both in breech presentation—to the operating theater. Dede speaks up calmly:

"Ain't dat woman convuhsing?"

I look over at the other woman in her first pregnancy who just arrived. She's lying on the bed by the window. Her teeth are clenched over her tongue, her arms are flexed and rigid and she's foaming at the mouth. Yeah, I'd call that a seizure. In fact, I'd call it eclampsia.

It was just five minutes go Dede told me the woman had a blood pressure of 160/100. I call for magnesium and an oral airway. The seizure has stopped by the time I get either. I still slip the curved plastic device over her tongue to keep her from biting her tongue or blocking her airway. The woman begins breathing easier immediately. By then, the magnesium has arrived. I give 2g slow IV push and ask Philip—who's come down from the nursing station to help—to put another 2g in the IV fluids.

Then I go do a routine c-section on the woman with breech-breech twins. Within a few minutest, I pull out two screaming babies with nice round heads, unsqueezed by any vicious attempt to be born vaginally.

I go downstairs while Mr. Wezzeh and Joseph clean up and get ready for the next c-section on the eclamptic lady. I see Gillian bent over a four year old boy.

"He was hit with a stick between his legs," Gillian answers my unspoken question. "Dr. Martin put in the foley catheter but there's no urine coming out."

She deflates the balloon on the catheter and reinserts it all the way. When clear urine comes out she re-inflates the balloon and sends the boy home.

"Do you want me to do the next c-section or do you?" I ask her.

"I'll do it."

"Ok, no problem..." and I fill her in on the details.

Then I get called outside for a steady stream of emergencies.

Two other pregnant women are in labor. A third one has premature rupture of membranes.

Then several cars of accident victims arrive. It was a multi-vehicle accident apparently. Most of the victims have just scratches and bruises. I tell them to take Paracetamol and Ibuprofen for the pain. I warn them that they'll feel worse tomorrow. They just need to rest and not panic.

One of the victims is pregnant. I do an ultrasound to make sure the baby is okay. Everything is normal except the baby is lying sideways (transverse lie). She walks out with some anti-inflammatories to go.

Her friend has a one centimeter cut on her forehead. I ask her caregiver to go buy me some superglue. He comes back in less than five minutes with an unopened tube. I pinch the skin to approximate it's edges and apply the superglue. Jerry is there and fans it with a chart to help the adhesive dry quicker. In a couple minutes the glue is hard and the wound well closed. I send her home.

I go up to labor and delivery. Gillian has just finished the c-section for the eclamptic patient. Gillian is now in the delivery room over the other first-time pregnancy girl who's sprawled on the floor. Gillian looks up as I walk in.

"Her pressure just went up quickly. Within minutes, she started seizing and fell of the exam table. We're getting her set up for another section." Two eclamptic patients in less than two hours!

Meanwhile, another car has arrived with two more victims from the same accident. The first has a couple of superficial scrapes. The second has a nasty 5cm gash on his left lower leg and a 2cm laceration on his right scalp.

I bring him into the treatment room and get ready to sew him up. Just as I'm getting set up, Otis calls me out for yet another patient in a car.

This is a young woman who is very pale and breathing heavy. The family states she always has heavy menses but she usually just takes blood tonic and is fine. This month, her period was extra heavy, though, and it lasted five days. I pull down her lower eyelid and it's white. She's severely anemic. She denies having vomiting, diarrhea or fever. I have R.B. bring her in.

Jeff is there and does the woman's hemoglobin. It's 3.6! Fortunately, the family has stayed around. I call for volunteers and have the first one come in to be tested to see if his blood type matches the patient's.

Meanwhile, Vivian has come down from upstairs and established an IV line. Normal Saline ins now running in full speed. The woman is thirsty. The older man with her, who I assume is her father, asks if he can bring her some water. I nod assent. He leaves and comes back quickly with a bag of water. She slurps half a bag down noisily.

At the same time, I'm injecting local anesthesia around the lacerations on the injured man's leg and scalp. Vivian speaks up.

"She vomit-tin'."

I look over and she's face down with her head hanging over the edge of the bed. Water is pouring out her mouth and nose. I turn back to my work. I keep hearing retching behind me. When I finish suturing I go over to look at her.

She's not breathing. I feel for a pulse. Nothing. Too late. I have Habakuk go tell Jeff to stop testing the family's blood and to have a family member come in. A short, stout girl in a miniskirt and heavy makeup comes in. I speak bluntly.

"She's dead."

The woman shrieks and runs down the hall. The man I just sutured couldn't walk. He had to be wheeled in on a wheelchair. I planned to admit him for observation. He pipes up.

"Doc, I wanna go home."

"Can you walk?"

"Yeah, I don' wanna be nex' to dis Ebola body..."

"It's not Ebola, she died from too much blood loss. Not every death is from Ebola, you know."

I can see in his eyes he's not convinced.

"But if you want to go home, no problem. We can give you some pills for the pain."

The formerly lame man almost jumps off the bed and runs out the door to wait in the lobby. Fear of Ebola can perform miracles!

An hour later, I'm in my office when Phillip, the security guard comes to see me. It appears the family of the dead girl have come to get the body. However, they want our staff to take her out of the hospital to them and put it in their vehicle. Our staff just want to give them gloves and have them take the body out themselves.

I go to the front door to try and mediate. I find that a small mob has gathered. There is a well dressed, good looking young man standing arrogantly in the center of the crowd. He has a look of astonishment on his face, like he's bewildered that he has to put up with lesser beings like the rest of us.

He's arguing with Vivian, who for some reason has come down off the wards and gone outside, just to be a part of the action. I call her in and tell her to get back up to work. This is not her business. I turn to the young ringleader.

"What's up?"

"We wan' to know how we shoul' get de body? We're not health care professionals. We don' know how to get a body. Can you lend us your materials and equipments so we can take de body out?" He speaks in an antagonistic way, in very proper English and obviously looking for a fight.

"Do I have to tell you how to pick up a body? Ok, try this: we'll give you gloves, then you come in and grab it like this..." and I mime grabbing something with both hands. "Then you carry it outside. You don't need to be a health professional to do that."

"But dat's what we're axing you, since you are health professionals. She die' under your care. You should know how to carry her out, so we're asking your staff to carry her out."

Every time I try to interrupt to explain something he cuts me off with a huff or a shrug or a look over his shoulder as if to say "see?" Then he keeps talking. I soon realize there is no reasoning with this man. But something stubborn and stupid inside me keeps me egging him on.

"Actually she didn't die under our care. You waited so long to bring her in that she actually died before we could start care on her. She was inside the hospital, it's true, but she didn't die under our care."

I might as well not have said anything because as soon as I start speaking he starts accusing me.

"You are hurting us inside with your words. Did you come here to huht us o' to help us? Huh, whahte man?"

I have to try and speak over him as he puffs himself up more and more in his righteous condemnation of us. His barrage of words doesn't let up.

"Look you insultin' us and turnin' us away and not lettin' us use de equipments you have readily available and how are we to know what to do wid a body..." He repeats over and over what he's said before.

I turn to Philip and Otis. "Look just close the gate..."

"Oh so you gonna lock us out? Since you've come we can't even dialogue. Before you got here, whahte man, we were dialoguin' nicely, but now you just shut us out like we nothin' and insult us..."

One of the women in their gang dares to move forward, "Le's jus' take ah sistuh an' go."

"Good idea, we'll get you gloves." I bring over a box and hand her a pair which she takes. But she's alone in her willingness to stand up to the sociopath bullying us and inciting the mob.

"Anyone else want gloves?" I offer holding out a pair.

No one steps forward. Soon the minor dictator has convinced even the one courageous friend to give back her gloves. They all get in their many nice new SUVs with their well dressed, cocky selves and drive off.

I don't suspect Ebola in this case, but I do suspect that what I've just witnessed might have something to do with why this epidemic looks like its wheeling more and more out of control every day.

I go back to my office and 15 minutes later our staff is decked out in protective gear carrying the woman's body on a stretcher out to the morgue. I go out and stop them.

"Why didn't you just do this before when those people were asking you to do it? We could've been done with the body. It would've been much less risk of contamination then you carrying the cadaver all the way down the stairs and out to the morgue. Not to mention the fact that someone else has to come get the body tomorrow from the morgue and who knows what else?"

Their sheepish glances make me realize I may have just stumbled on another clue to the persistence of Ebola epidemic this time around in West Africa. Is there any hope it will ever end?

Excision

September 17

I'm exhausted. I tossed and turned all last night. I'm not sure why. Maybe the stress. Yesterday was long and filled with difficult decisions: does this person have Ebola or not? If I turn them away they'll probably die. If I admit them and they have Ebola, I or the staff may die.

Not to mention the stress of having so many sick inpatients and emergency patients. It probably didn't help that I read a lot of articles late on the internet late at night about how the Ebola crisis is worsening, Obama's sending in the US Military, WHO needs a billion dollars to fight it, etc.

Whatever the case, I certainly couldn't sleep, my thoughts were racing and I could feel my stomach in knots. I tried prostrating myself, praying, crying, stretching, anything and everything I knew to relieve stress, but nothing worked.

When dawn mercifully breaks, I head up to my office. I barely arrive and Phillip comes to get me.

"Emuhjuncy in de cah. OB payshunt."

I put on gloves, walk down the hallway and outside the front door. A obviously pregnant woman is waiting there in a beat-up yellow taxi. She says she's nine months pregnant and been in labor for five days. She went to a health center yesterday afternoon and her waters broke at 5pm last night.

This morning, the people at the health center referred her here to Cooper Hospital. She hands me the referral slip where it states she's fully dilated but has obstructed labor.

I ask her about headache, cough, sore throat, fever, chills, vomiting, diarrhea and bleeding. Of course, she says "no" to all of the above. Everyone knows that those are screening questions for Ebola. So you better say "no" or they'll turn you away. However, I feel Ebola is unlikely so I admit her to the maternity ward.

I have her follow me down the hall, up the stairs and then down the half flight of stairs into the dimly let labor and delivery room. A bare wooden table with a hole in one end holding a plastic basin awaits. It's been covered with a couple of thin operating table pads and then a small piece of plastic sheet.

The midwives gear up in their hazardous waste disposal gear with full body suits, boots, double gloves, masks and hats. I also put one on but it's too short for my long legs and arms. I pull on some extra long gynecologic gloves that cover my wrists but my ankles are left exposed. I cover my crocs with a couple of OR shoe covers that are more symbolic than useful.

As I examine the woman, I notice that she has been excised. Female circumcision is practiced frequently here. While I've heard certain tribes in Chad also perform the ritual, I've only seen one woman who's been excised in my ten years there. She happened to be a Christian. None of the Muslim women I've examined in Chad have been circumcised.

Here in predominantly Christian Liberia, though, practically all the women have had their clitoris surgically removed in their prepubertal years. Unfortunately, I'm sure anesthesia was not a big part of the process.

It seems many people associate female circumcision with Islam and use it to promote anti-Muslim sentiment. In my experience, limited though it may be to two countries, it's Christians that are doing it more than Muslims. Not that I think it is either a Christian or a Muslim practice. It's rather part of the syncretism that characterizes those two religions here in Africa. Most West, Central and North Africans are still animists and traditionalists,. Many have just added either Christianity or Islam to their existing beliefs.

What I have also noticed, is having a previous excision leads to a lot more complications during vaginal deliveries. Two of the five women I've done symphysiotomies on have had large and deep periurethral tears. The scar tissue from the circumcision is stiff and doesn't stretch with descent of the fetal head like normal, unbrutalized tissue does. Instead of expanding, the scar just tears, leaving a painful wound that is difficult to repair.

This patient in front of me is completely dilated. The fetal head is severely deformed like a cone head, a condition called caput. She needs a symphysiotomy. I numb up the skin and subcutaneous tissues all the way down to the symphysis pubis. I ask Dede to insert a foley catheter.

"It won' go i'," Dede complains after a few failed attempts at insertion.

We team up. I push hard with both hands on the fetal head in between contractions. This relieves the obstruction on the urethra and Dede manages to get the foley in. I pause to pray before slicing down quickly to the cartilage between the pelvic bones. I insert my other hand inside to displace the foley and it's concomitant urethra to one side. Having my hand inside also helps me judge the depth of how far to incise without damaging internal tissues. I saw through the cartilage.

"Pull the legs down and out," I order my two assistants as I insert a finger into the symphysiotomy wound. When the gap between the pelvic bones reaches 2 cm I have my assistants stop. I open up an oxytocin drip and a couple minutes later the woman has strong contractions and starts to push.

I inject lidocaine into the right lateral inferior vulva and cut an episiotomy. After my previous experience with severe tears on excised woman, I feel this could help to prevent that complication. This will enlarge the vaginal opening enough to get the large fetal head out even if the superior tissues can't stretch.

Sure enough, the baby comes out a minute later with no tears. He's huge, cone-headed and screams easily. I repair the symphysiotomy and episiotomy wounds.

I go upstairs to start the day with inpatient rounds.

Steve

September 18

I'm walking down the hall and Tom approaches me with a chart. Tom is amazing. He literally lives in the hospital 24/7. He works in billing but also turns the generator on and off, makes sure the water tank is filled, and a million other little things. He goes home for a few hours every day when things are calm but can be called back and there in a few minutes.

"Dis man goin' home?" Tom asks.

I look over the chart and see it's for Steve, the 18 year old with the left femur fracture. I'm annoyed. I had just called up John Fankhauser at ELWA to see if we could use their SIGN instruments. They don't have the target arm I'm used to, but I figure something is better than nothing. I knew with any more delay in surgery the family would want to take him home to the traditional bone setter. I'm supposed to see John in an hour to talk over the details and now Steve wants to go home?

I go upstairs and down to M5, Steve's room. He's lying comfortably in bed playing with his smart phone. He obviously has no pain. His leg is in traction and out to length...although I see that it has internally rotated a bit. I'll need to fix that. I make a mental note.

"Steve, what's up?"

"Fine," he looks up and smiles.

"I've got good news. We found the instruments we need so we can do your surgery either today or tomorrow. Good thing you didn't leave last week."

He smiles and nods. I feel reassured and go back downstairs. Within a few minutes Dr. Sonii, Mrs. Carter and Gillian all come into my office. Steve's uncle and Grandmother are with them. The uncle seems educated, but the grandmother barely speaks English through her almost toothless mouth.

I'm reminded of a line by Jeff Foxworthy: "If you've ever been accused of lying through your TOOTH....you might be a redneck." He also says he's found "rednecks everywhere" and I'm sure I'm seated across from a Liberian redneck right now.

The uncle listens to us explain why we want to keep Steve and do the surgery. He nods and agrees. But the Granny just scowls and then speaks up, spitting and yelling in her dialect. The uncle translates into Liberian English.

"She say she wanna ta' de boy home."

We question them and explain to them more about the benefits and risks. Grandma insists through her translator that Steve needs to see the traditional bone setter. This healer will apply the appropriate seven leaves from the city and five leaves from the bush and wrap it well. Her other grandson, Steve's older brother also had a broken leg. He was treated by this man and is now playing soccer with no problems.

"Who de he' o' de family heeuh?" Asks Dr. Sonii.

The uncle replies that he is acting as Steve's father. He's the responsible one.

"Way I seein' it de gramma de head...we jus' gotta le' em go," concludes Dr. Sonii.

"We can't just give in so easily..." I start to argue.

"Listen to me," interrupts Mrs. Carter. "I know dese people. I live' wi' dem sevuhnteeeen yeauhs an' i' won' make any differuhnce wi' dem. We can talk all day, dey gonna take hi' home. We gotte jus' let em go."

Gillian also agrees with Mrs. Carter and Dr. Sonii. Despite my huge frustration at being barely thwarted in my desire to appropriately manage Steve's fracture, I have to concede defeat. I nod grudgingly.

When the uncle translates our decision to the toothless Liberian redneck, her scowl changes instantly to a huge grin. She has beaten us! She gets up and goes down the hall. She'd be dancing a jig...if she could. That's when I notice she's limping. One leg shorter is than the other and twisted out. I can't help but ask Dr. Sonii:

"Do you think she went to see the same traditional bone setter for her leg?"

"Probably," says Dr. Sonii with a his half smile as he turns to the uncle who hasn't left yet. "At fuhst I tought you was de head o de family but I see you incapable of standin' up to de woman."

He continues to politely insult the man as the man smiles and nods, emasculated in the face of the fearsome redneck grandma. He trots off after her while Gillian and I go upstairs.

Gillian has brought the old power drill from accounting (don't ask me why they have it). Alex brings Betadine. I detach the weights and cord from the traction pin. I swab the skin and pin with the iodine scrub. Gillian gives Steve Diazepam and Tramadol injectins. I attach the drill to the pin. I put the drill in reverse and in five seconds the pin is out. Steve lies on the bed with a silly grin on his face. I turn and walk out, rabid.

I never see him again.

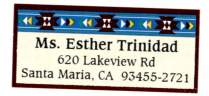

Abortion
September 19

Jerry takes me aside the next morning.

"Doctuh, dat woman las' naht, de family not tellin' de truf. I work wi' MSF lon' tahm ago an' we see dese women tryun' to ha' abortions all de tahm. Dey stick tings up insahd, o' dey take herbs fra' de witsh doctuh, dey no' tellin' de truf."

Apparently, the family of the girl who died last night from vaginal hemorrhage is at the hospital this morning. They claim they didn't know anything about their daughter's illness. Nor did they know that their daughter was dead.

The mob from last night was not family, but "friends." And the man who brought her was not her father but a "doctor." That's why Jerry suspects that the doctor botched the abortion, knew she was in trouble and brought her here with a story of heavy menses to throw us off his scent, hoping we could work a miracle and save her life. Unfortunately, we were fresh out of miracles last night.

"Jerry, I think you're right. Good call." I go back to work.

In a few hours, I get called out to see a woman in the back seat of a taxi.

"What's happening?" I inquire.

The husband explains. "Yestuhday, she fell. She tree o' fo' month pregnant an' now she bleedin'."

She does look anemic with pale conjunctiva and rapid, shallow respirations.

"Bring her in," I say.

The woman, Dao, is brought in to the Emergency Room. Vivian and Habakuk help me start a couple of IV lines and get some fluid boluses going. Jeff comes in and checks her hemoglobin which is 6 g/dl. I order two units of packed red blood cells to be transfused tonight.

Three family members are still here. I hope at least a couple will be able to donate. I tell the husband to call more relatives. I pull out the ultrasound. I want to make sure she doesn't have an ectopic pregnancy. I confirm an intrauterine fetal demise with the amniotic sac at the internal cervical os. I also see evidence of separation of the placenta anteriorly. We need to do a D&C. But I need blood first.

We get one unit. The two other relatives are disqualified by wrong blood type or Hepatitis B. I wait all afternoon and no other family members show up. Finally, it's evening and they can't come because of the curfew. A hemoglobin of 6 isn't super critical and her bleeding is only spotty currently. I decide she can wait for her D&C until tomorrow when the family can come and give more blood.

The next morning, the family still hasn't come. I decide to just do the D&C. Dorbor, the anesthetist comes and gets me.

"De hemoglobin 6 or 3.1?"

I look at the chart and see that the nurse had ordered another hemoglobin later last night. The result came back 3.1 g/dl. No one bothered to tell me. After confirming with the lab's log book that it really was done on Dao, I feel we really need more blood before we can safely do the operation.

One unit just won't cut it with a hemoglobin of 3. Who knows how much she'll bleed during the curettage? I start asking around for volunteers. The inpatient pharmacist says she's willing to give because she has a hemoglobin of 14 and she thinks that's too high. She's already started taking Chloramphenicol tablets to help her "reduce her blood"! I explain why that's a really bad idea and if she really wants to lower her hemoglobin, donating blood is much safer and more useful.

She agrees but says I need to give her some juice.

I go downstairs, find the husband and tell him to buy me two cartons of juice. I start asking the staff downstairs and most refuse. Finally, Robert, one of the drivers who speaks French after spending several years in Ivory Coast, agrees.

"Pas de problème, docteur," Robert says with a big grin.

Dao's husband comes back with one carton of juice which I give to Robert.

"Hey man, we need more juice," I tell the husband.

He soon comes back with another carton in a blue plastic bag. I take it to the pharmacist who is already pumping her blood into a blood bag lying on the lab floor.

At last, I'm ready to do the D&C. The woman is placed in the lithotomy position. Dorbor gives her Ketamine. I insert the vaginal retractors and meet a foul smelling mass of half rotting placenta. A clear amniotic sac with a 4 cm long fetus inside follows the placenta. The baby has obviously been dead for several days.

I pull out the chunks of decaying flesh with a ring forceps until I find the open cervix. I grasp the anterior lip with the ring forceps and pull it up and out. The cervix has a couple areas of greenish black necrosis. I curette inside the uterus, scraping off nasty chunks of left over placenta and products of conception.

Thankfully, she hardly bleeds at all. She starts to contract her abdominal and leg muscles as she emerges from dissociative anesthesia. Her legs close and she scoots up on the bed making it impossible to finish the D&C.

"Some Diazepam, maybe?" I calmly ask Dorbor who obliges rapidly.

The woman is soon able to be repositioned and I finish the case. She gets the three bags of blood in short order. In the evening, another relative comes and she gets a fourth unit.

The next day, she is looking great, breathing normally and has no bleeding. I just have one question to ask:

"Ma'am, you tried to get rid of the pregnancy at home didn't you?" She gives me a blank stare and looks at Philip, the nurse for translation.

"Yo' trahd to abort de baby a' home yeah?" Dao looks sheepish and starts to deny...

"It wasn't a question, but more of a statement," I say with a half smile. "You can't fool your doctor..."

She looks down with a sly grin.

"It's dangerous," I continue. "You almost died..."

I walk out.

* * * * *

I've been called outside for another obstetrical emergency. The woman looks small and very pregnant. She presents a referral slip from a health center. This is her third pregnancy and she's had two c-sections previously. Looking at her, I'm guessing that the scientific indication was "big baby, small mommy."

I take her upstairs to Labor and Delivery. Right before the door I see one of the larger staff members sitting on a chair. I don't bother to look closer to identify who it is until I enter labor and delivery. There's no one. The woman outside must be the midwife. I have the patient wait inside the delivery room. I go back and approach the midwife.

She's crying.

"What's going on?" I ask.

"R. B., you know, de gir' dat work downstairs sometahm, dey say she jus' die o' Ebola."

"What? Are you sure? I was just told that she went to JFK to be tested, but that she wasn't that sick. Are you sure she's dead?"

"Dats wha' dey sayin," and she bursts into sobs.

I want to comfort her, but no touching is the rule in the Ebola Capital of te World. Even a pat on the back is off limits.

"I'm sorry," I mumble. "I'm going to go confirm with Dr. Sonii."

I go downstairs and find Dr. Sonii in Mrs. Carter's office. A tall, serious looking man is talking to Gillian. Gillian is explaining why she wants the man's wife to go get tested for Ebola. The man himself works for the Ebola task force at JFK Hospital. He should be able to pull some strings to get her in quickly to be tested.

He nods, "I'll go trah an' get an ambewlance to take huh in."

After the man leaves, I ask Dr. Sonii about R.B..

"No, no!" He retorts. "Dats jus' a rumuh. I jus' talk wi' ma colleague a' JFK who workin' wi' de Ebola cases. He jus' started an IV on huh and huh test still pending."

I feel relieved. At the same time, I can't help but wonder who exposed her? Everyone is saying it was the small boy we couldn't find an IV on. Apparently his dad died of Ebola a short time later. A few days after being discharged, the boy died too.

I spent some time finding a femoral IV line on him. While I was wearing gloves, who knows how much exposure I had? Did I touch him accidentally? A few groups are speculating that while the major route of contamination is through contact, some airborne transmission of Ebola is possible.

I've been having a headache all day. It's been getting worse the last two nights since I haven't slept well. Now I'm feeling kind of nauseated too. Do I have Ebola? I don't have a fever, but now I'm not so sure that's a guarantee.

I feel the need to get away. I've been on the compound for five days without leaving. I go find Gillian and ask for the keys to the car. I throw in the surfboard and head out to Oddny Beach.

It's been raining and storming heavily the past three days and even though it's sunny this afternoon, the wind is still up. I don't expect much from the surf. But I need to get some exercise, even if it means paddling around in choppy seas.

I turn down the road towards the beach, cross the speed bumps, pass the guard house in the middle of the road, motor past the hotel to the right and pull around to my favorite parking spot under the palm tree. There is a nice lawn with umbrella covered tables at an outdoor cabana going right up to the beach.

I glance out over the ocean and see gorgeous, glassy sets lining up not to far from the beach. While the peaks are not consistent, there are some nice curls peeling alternately left or right. NO WAY!

I quickly take of my crocs and t-shirt, zip the car keys in the side pocket of my shorts, attach the surfing leash to my right ankle and dash down the sand. I plunge through the breakers, dive over a wave and start paddling like mad to make it out past the break.

It turns into an exhausting session with some excellent, if short beach break rides. I just wish I had a more maneuverable board instead of this learner's soft top. But beggars can't be choosers. And I'm certainly having fun!

Finally, wasted, I catch a last wave in. I ride it almost to the beach where the previous wave comes rushing back to clash with my wave and send me sprawling. I recover and lunge towards the sand. The undertow tries to pull me back out as the waves try and pound me into the beach. I'm winded, breathing heavy and my arms are limp. But I have no headache and my nausea is gone.

Maybe surfing is the vaccine we've all been looking for against Ebola!

Fever

September 20

I'm just coming back from a pleasant evening with Dr. John and Gillian at the Sajj Restaurant. We've just gone outside to get in John's car when my phone rings.

"Hello?"

"Yeah dis de nuhse a' de hospital, Coopuh Hospital, dere a wuhmuhn wi' twin' de fuhst she born a' home, an' de secuhnd nah' bohn…" followed by a lot more real Liberian English I don't understand.

"Ok, fine, I'm not far, I'll be right there…"

I hear a lot more gibberish on the other end. I hang up. We get in the car and John drives us back to the Hospital. We've just turned onto 12th Street and are about a block from the hospital when I get another call. It's only been a couple minutes since the last one.

"Hello?"

I hear more incomprehensible Liberian English. I think I know the nurse who's calling me…I can never understand her!.

"I'm coming…two seconds," I reply as I hang up.

We're at the hospital. There's a station wagon outside. Inside is a woman lying across the back seat. She's delivered a dead baby already and the second one isn't coming. I check her temperature with the infrared thermometer: 38.9 C. Not good.

I examine her conjunctiva. They're pale. No increased redness for sure. I look in her mouth for signs of dehydration and bleeding. Everything appears normal. It still could be early Ebola, but it's probably malaria. In any case, we have to get the second baby out. I have the nurse bring her upstairs.

I put on the long gynecologic gloves and examine the woman. The first umbilical cord is hanging limply outside the vulva. Inside, I feel the second amniotic sac intact with what feels like either a foot or a hand bouncing against the bulging membrane.

I examine her uterus from the abdominal side. The fetus seems vertically oriented, meaning it's probably a foot presentation and not a hand or transverse lie. I rupture her membranes and amniotic fluid shoots out.

I see that a few drops have got on my scrubs and on my left croc. I quickly get some water in a basin and add some chlorine. I soak the stains on my scrubs with the mixture. I dump the rest over my crocs. My feet are swimming in diluted bleach. I pull on a full protective gown, a face mask with a shield, and two layers of gloves including a long gynecologic pair.

I go back to the woman and see two tiny feet sticking out. I grab them in my left hand and pull. The baby moves down well until his shoulders get stuck. I reach in and swing the anterior arm down and out. I twist the fetal body rapidly and deliver the second arm which is now anterior.

I put my finger in the baby's mouth and pull the chin down to the chest. I place gentle traction on the feet that are still gripped in my left hand. The head isn't coming out. I apply stronger traction. Nothing.

Finally, I release the feet, grab the baby around the pelvis and really pull strong and steady. The head pops out in a gush of meconium-stained amniotic fluid. The baby has great tone and looks like he wants to scream. I quickly suction out this mouth and nose. I clamp and cut the cord. By the time I get him to the table he's screaming his little lungs out.

The placenta quickly follows and the uterus is rock hard. There are no tears and minimal bleeding. I take off my suit and go home. On entering, I immediately take off all my clothes and dump them in a large basin. I fill it with water and Rexguard, some kind of local antiseptic. I take a quick bucket shower, sloshing water all over me with a tin cup. Then I soap up and rinse off again. I go to sleep.

What seems like only a few minutes later, I hear the buzz of the the door alarm in my bedroom. I go out to the living room and look out the window.

"What?"

"Doctuh, dere a wuhmuhn wi' IUFD. De hea' out between huh legs. We gi' huh pit but de hea' still dere." It's Dede, our best midwife.

"How long ago?"

"Fo' howuhs."

"Four hours? Where is she?"

"Downstehuhs, she got feevuh. 39 degree."

"I'm coming."

I pull on my scrubs and crocs, grab my office keys and lock the house door behind me. In my office, I pull out a bag of protective gear. Fever means she could have Ebola. And it's going to be messy. I put on two pairs of gloves and an apron over the monkey suit. I top it off with a mask and face shield. I enter the holding room across from our injection room we call the "Emergency." The woman is stark naked lying on a regular exam table. There is a fat, deformed fetal head sticking out between her legs face up. The face is mottled and red, the skin starting to desquamate.

I pull her down to the end of the bed. Dede has put on her PPE as well so I have her hold the woman's legs in the lithotomy position. I pull down with all my strength on the head. The anterior shoulder is stuck and won't budge: a shoulder dystocia. It's only the second I've ever seen and the second in less than a week!

I feel around inside to see if I can rotate the shoulder out from under the pelvic bone. No deal. I find the posterior shoulder and am able to get my index finger under the armpit. The posterior shoulder slowly slides out. I put traction on the head and deliver the anterior shoulder.

The dead baby comes out in a gush of meconium-stained amniotic fluid and dark blood. There's a red trash can at the edge of the bed. The baby falls directly in the bucket still connected by the umbilical cord to the placenta which is still attached to the mother's uterus.

"Instruments!"

Dede hands me clamps and scissors. The baby is soon detached from the placenta.

"Hold the trash can!" I ask Dede.

I then put traction on the placenta. It soon separates and plops on top of the dead baby. Then the woman starts bleeding like stink. I try uterine massage but it's super floppy. Blood keeps streaming out.

"Oxytocin!...Quickly!" Dede runs off and soon comes back with two ampoules which she injects.

"Erogmetrine!" I shout.

The bleeding hasn't slowed and the uterus still hasn't contracted. Blood is flowing off the bed. Half falls in the trash can. The other half is coagulating quickly on the floor in a puddle of bloody jello.

Dede injects the Ergometrine in her thigh while I continue to massage the uterus to no avail.

"I need an 18 gauge catheter and some Saline!" Vivian has come down and goes back up to get supplies. She comes back with a foley catheter, a urine bag and an 18 gauge IV cannula. No IV fluids. And she's not wearing any protective gear.

"Get your gown on! This is dangerous! Don't come in here like that!" She quickly leaves and comes back appropriately dressed with the IV fluids. Meanwhile, the bleeding hasn't stopped. The uterus is still floppy even though I'm squeezing it between an internal hand and an external one.

"Two more ampoules of Oxytocin and some more Ergometrine!" Dede has to run back upstairs and comes back what seems like hours later.

Finally, the uterus firms up. I clear out the last blood clots and go pick up the IV cannula. I put a glove as a tourniquet around the patient's biceps. Thankfully I feel a decent vein on her forearm. I soon have a good IV running with a Normal Saline bolus.

Dede puts 20 more units of Oxytocin in the drip which is running wide open. I start cleaning up. I dump diluted chlorine water over all the blood spots. I pick up the clots with toilet paper. Then I douse it all with more bleach solution. I collect all the materials we've used, dump them over the baby in the trash can, and drown it all in the disinfecting solution.

I strip off my protective gear after dousing it in chlorine water. I wash my hands in chlorine water up to my elbows and dump some more on my crocs. I go home, strip down naked and repeat the earlier ritual of washing and disinfecting my scrubs. I take another bucket shower. By this time it's 5:00 AM.

Time to get ready for my day off. I'm going to Robertsport to check out it's legendary left point break. Robert and Abraham are supposed to accompany me.

We'll see if they show up.

Paradise

September 21

I've just finished delivering the dead baby who came in with its head stuck between the mother's legs. I make my last minute preparations to go to Robertsport. I drive Gillian's Honda CRV outside and lock the gate to the compound behind me. I look up and see Robert's tall, lanky frame waiting outside the hospital with a big grin on his face.

"Abbie nous attend en ville. On y va..." Robert spent years in Ivory Coast so he likes to keep up on his French with me. He hops in the passenger seat and we head through the broken streets of Monrovia to pick up Abraham on the other side of town.

The roads are mostly empty on this Sunday morning which makes what could be a horn-filled traffic jam congested trip pass rapidly. Abraham waves us down outside a little shop near the big port warehouses. He's wearing a bright orange shirt as if to make sure we don't miss him.

We are soon out of the chaos of Monrovia and into the bush. Jungle foliage stretches as far as the eye can see, creeping over mountains, down ravines and up to the edge of the many large rivers we cross on bridges. Here and there, a farmer has made a heroic effort to wrench some order out of the forest. But the creeping things of the jungle invade even what originally must have been orderly orchards of oil palms.

There is one brief police checkpoint with cones blocking the road. The female officer lifts a cone and waves us through with a smile. We come up to the turn off for Robertsport and there's a rope stretched across between two guardhouses. A policeman comes up.

"Yo' gotta ge' out de cah an' wash yo' hands," he informs us nonchalantly. "Den we take yo' temperatshure."

We nod in agreement and the rope is lowered. The smiling officer points the infrared temperature gun at my temple and says:

"32.5! Yoo good ta go."

"I think your thermometer is broken," I offer. "I'd be almost dead if my temperature was really only 32."

"Maybe yo' need tuh change de battereees!" says Robert with a huge smile.

"Tank you vehhhhhyyy much!" the officer exclaims.

After we wash our hands in chlorine water, the cop waves goodbye as we turn left towards Robertsport. The road stays paved for a short distance and then turns to laterite. If it was regularly graded, it probably would be a decent road.

However, years of neglect have left it ridden with potholes. They slow our progress dramatically. After several miles, we come upon a huge inland sea to the right. It's glassy and laps up the the edge of the road through some mangrove trees. Soon, the water is coming up to the left side of the road too. It seems like the road is actually a land bridge.

We wind up and down some steep grades on the side of a small mountain. We top a hill and see Robertsport spread below us. The town is quaint, looking more like a caribbean sea town then an African village. I can see slivers of beach jutting out to a narrow channel that separates the inland sea from the huge bay spread out below us.

The sun is shining, the water is reflecting and I can see glassy faced waves beckoning. We wander around a bit, asking questions until we finally get pointed in the right direction. After a steep descent down a laterite grade, we find ourselves in some kind of campground with ancient, Vietnam war era army tents in groves of huge shade trees almost up to the water's edge. To the left is a forest of massive Cottonwood trees, some dozens of feet in diameter and hundreds of feet high.

As I wander through the shade of the Cottonwoods after defecating in the bush, a young boy comes up to me. He introduces himself as Samuel, the reigning junior surf champion of Liberia.

"We go' fahve point breayks heyuh," He states proudly. "We go' a surf club an' 50 bohds o'so. Dey wa' dese to' whahte men teachin' surf lessuhns."

"Which is the best break today?" I interject.

"I tink Shipwrecks. Dis one heyuh, I' front o' us? Dis numbuh two, den tree, fo' an de fif' one, dat Shipwrecks." He points past some already inviting, glassy waves peeling left off various slick black rock formations.

I decide to try the closest point break. It's ight in front of us peeling left off a jumble of black boulders jutting out from the beach and then into a small cove.

Ebola-iculous

I paddle out and as I'm waiting for the next set to roll through, I look back at the beach in time to see a strange sight: Abbie is prancing in the shore break like a native american doing a war dance around a bonfire. Robert streaking away from me down the beach stark naked and arms flailing.

And I thought I was the only one having a good time!

I catch a few small peelers but as the tide comes in it's looking better a little farther up. I paddle around the boulders and into the second cove with a huge rock sticking out in the middle of it. The waves are breaking near the rock but it looks like if you catch one it'll peel around without crashing you into it.

I paddle up to where they have been breaking and wait. It seems I've struck out again. I continue on to the next break which is along the edge of the cove. There is a scattering of shiny ebony rocks strewn haphazardly along the beach and out into the water where a small pyramid shaped one hovers near the take off point.

I'm a little nervous and let a few sets roll in before I find one that's breaking a little farther off the pyramid rock. I find myself on a fat, glassy shoulder pushing me into the cove. Unfortunately, my soft top beginner board is completely unmaneuverable. So I just glide along. But I'm not complaining! The conditions are perfect and I spend about four hours in the water without a break.

Little by little I'm joined by some of the local Liberian surfers. The first out is Morris. He quickly shows me that he's on his home turf catching wave after wave close to the pyramid rock and shredding them with a wry smile on his face.

Then comes out the second Samuel and Prince. A couple of other surfers are also out but don't introduce themselves. There's only one thing missing: a rabid, territorial, competitive spirit that dominates so many other surfing spots around the globe, especially in the USA.

But then again, I wonder how the Liberians would react if it wasn't just one weekend warrior who descended on their secret break, but a whole mob of wannabe surfers?

I take a break out of sheer exhaustion. The car is parked under a shade tree right on the beach. Robert is talking with a local girl and Abbie is asleep in the driver's seat. I grab a huge slice of local bread and slather it with gobs of peanut butter and jelly. I have two sandwiches along with a liter and a half of water. Prince comes up to talk.

"Can I bohrow yo' bohd? Catch a wa' o' two?"

I hesitate for a second, after all it's not my board. But then, throwing caution to the wind and embracing the vibe of the place and the moment, I give in.

"Sure man, tear it up."

Prince runs off eagerly and is soon paddling out into the lineup. Apparently, his brother Alfred is the three time reigning Liberian surfing champion. He has traveled to Sierra Leone and Nigeria representing his country. Unfortunately, he's developed a drug habit and had to be disqualified in one competition for smoking in between heats.

I watch Prince catch a few waves. Either he's not even close to as good as his brother or my board isn't made for these conditions. Whatever the case, he's struggling a little. However, you'd never guess it by the smile on his face when he finally comes in.

I go back out and catch a few more long rides at the first point I surfed. It has now picked up again. I start to feel the salt burning my stomach, face, and back. I'm sunburned! I've never been sunburned before in 10 years in Africa! My arms are also becoming like lead weights. I catch a couple of small rides, waiting for that last big one to come in as my last ride. It never comes. I settle for a mediocre wave and ride it to the beach.

Robert has taken the car to go by fish for Dr. Sonii and Mrs. Carter. Abbie is resting under a shade tree. I join him and my skin thanks me. The trip back to Monrovia is uneventful as I sleep most of the way in the back seat while Robert drives like a maniac.

I certainly never expected to come to Liberia and have such an unreal, exotic experience. I came to join the fight against Ebola. But come to think of it, that's just the kind of thing God would do: hide Paradise deep in the heart of the Ebola Capital of the World!

Closed!
September 22

It was too good to be true. SDA Cooper was the only hospital in Monrovia to be open during the whole Ebola epidemic thus far. And we were the only hospital without Ebola casualties among its staff.

This morning, I get called into a meeting in Mrs. Carter's office. Dr. Martin, Dr. Sonii, Steve, Gillian, the Chaplain and Mrs. Carter are all present.

I learn that R.B., the ER nurse's aide who took herself to JFK Hospital last week to get tested for Ebola has been confirmed Ebola positive. She has had early treatment, which is a good prognostic indicator. But the ongoing treatment is dependent on Steve taking money, medicines and supplies over to JFK every day and bribing the hospital staff to take care of R.B. She's conscious, but has started having bloody diarrhea.

No one has heard from Aaron either. He's one of the cleaning staff. He's been sick for over a week, taking malaria medicines at home. He refuses to come to come to Cooper Hospital, go get tested for Ebola or even let anyone see him. He's been having rectal bleeding. He claims it's his hemorrhoids, but he won't let anyone examine him. He lives by himself.

Steve went to visit him yesterday and found his door locked. No one answered his loud banging. Gillian had told me earlier that the rumor is circulating that someone found him dead with his pupils fixed and dilated. This apparently hasn't been confirmed. Someone plans to go break down Aaron's door and find out.

As a result, yesterday no midwives or nurses showed up to work during the day and only one nurse came at night. Today, there's one nurse and one midwife on duty, as well as the Outpatient Department staff.

Steve confirms that many nurses and midwives have called him to say they're not coming in. They're too afraid. Many of them had contact with R.B. or with the same patients she did. As a result, they are frightened and don't want to come to the hospital. Steve recommends that we temporarily close down. Everyone seems to be in agreement. After a brief discussion, we decide to close for three weeks. The time will serve as a sort of quarantine since that is the incubation period for Ebola.

As of tomorrow, we aren't seeing patients. If you're pregnant and need to deliver? Malaria, anemic and need a blood transfusion? Surgical emergency? Sorry, find someplace else…if you can. And chances are, you're on your own as none of the other hospitals in town are taking new patients.

Gillian and I and whatever nurses are willing to help will take care of the current inpatients until they are discharged. We only have six left since Gillian discharged many today. Tomorrow, we'll do the last operation on Titus to close his colostomy. He should be able to go home in 2-3 days.

By Friday, the SDA Cooper Hospital will be completely shut down.

* * * * *

Later in the morning, Bendu calls me to go see Mr. Wennie. Mrs. Wennie is helping him stumble into his office. I follow them and see Mr. Wennie sitting in a chair. He has an obvious right facial droop and is complaining that his left arm "not feel raht."

"His preshuh 150 ower 100, doctuh," says Bendu.

"Did he take his pressure medicine this morning?" I ask Mrs. Wennie.

"No, he didna take it."

I have her bring his meds. I give them to Mr. Wennie to swallow along with four baby aspirins. He can barely swallow. One pill rests on his outer lip and he chokes on the water. It's looking more and more like a stroke. I go get a thing of yoghurt from my fridge and bring it to him. He swallows that fine with the rest of his tablets. We lay him down on a mattress behind his desk. I ask Bendu to bring some oxygen. We'll see what happens.

Mrs. Wennie comes back a half hour later to tell me Mr. Wennie has refused the oxygen. I go into his office. His facial droop is gone and he's sitting at his desk without oxygen. He's talking better but says his left arm still doesn't feel right. I speak firmly with him about the need for oxygen and he finally lays down again and lets us put the oxygen on.

I go back to my office.

Ebola-iculous

Phillip calls me to come see another "emuhguhncy in de cah'." A woman is in the back seat. She had a stroke three weeks ago. She went to a clinic, was diagnosed with "presshuh" and given a water tablet which she took for a few days, then stopped.

Later, she went to a Chinese medical clinic. She shows me a bag filled with bottles labeled in Chinese and baggies of black pellets. Since yesterday evening she has been having right sided seizures. I tell them there's nothing we can really do except for comfort care. I send them home with some pain and sleep tablets.

I take off my gloves and wash my hands in chlorine water before going back into the hospital. Before I can get inside, a man comes up holding a sick seven year old girl in his arms. She is semi-conscious, but otherwise looks healthy. Her temperature is normal. The man explains that she had a headache last night with fever and then convulsed this morning. I admit her for treatment of cerebral malaria.

As I go back to my office, I realize suddenly that this may be the last patient I ever admit to the SDA Cooper Hospital.

I can't tell if I'm relieved or sad...

Limbo

September 23

    I have a lot of dreams. All of them involve Cooper Hospital in some way. I don't remember anything distinct: just images of patients, surgeries, deliveries, staff, life, etc. I get up often to drink water. I'm thirsty. I wake up after 6:00AM and make breakfast since I know the generator will be off around 7:30AM. With nothing happening at the hospital, there may be no power all day. I cook on a little hot plate so if I want food, it better be now.

    After a massive bowl of oatmeal I lay around on the couch awhile, listen to some music and reflect. I just can't help feeling sad that we're closed. But then again, we're really not. Not yet. I get up and go up to the wards to see the remaining inpatients.

    There's a woman here in labor since yesterday. With no midwife and no nurse overnight nothing has been done for her. I start an IV, give her some antibiotics and start a Pitocin drip. She has been at 5-6cm dilatation with weak contractions since yesterday's admission.

    It's her second pregnancy and she says she's been leaking water since yesterday evening. I lay my hand on her abdomen to measure the strength of her contractions. With just a tiny bit of Pit, she starts really wincing. The uterus firms up well under my palm, yet still relaxes after less than a minute.

    Within 5 minutes, the woman speaks up: "I wanna toilet."

    I quickly examine her and her cervix is now 8 cm dilated! I quickly fumble for a full body suit, pull on shoe covers, get some of the long gyn gloves and put on a face mask with eye shield. None too soon!

    I re-examine her and the head is coming down. She's completely dilated! She starts to push and within a few minutes a grimacing, flexing 4.5kg man child is yelling at the world, his mouth wide open in shock at this brutal welcome to life. I rub him all over to dry him, suction his mouth and then wrap him in a brightly colored African pattern cloth.

I open up the Pitocin drip and the uterus firms up under my hand. A gush of dark blood comes and with gentle traction on the cord the placenta comes out easily. Within seconds the woman is up, getting her clothes back on and packing her things. I've taken the boy out to his waiting dad and the woman goes to postpartum on her own two feet.

I clean up the mess, dropping the placenta in a plastic bag lining a metal bucket and wiping upall the blood, meconium and amniotic fluid with a chlorine drenched OR towel. I carefully take off my protective gear and put it in the red hazardous waste can.

I then prepare the next patient for surgery. She's HIV positive with a breech presentation at term. She was scheduled for a c-section tomorrow, but with the "closure" of the hospital, we decide to do it today. Hopefully she can be sent home by Friday.

Gillian wants to do the anesthesia. I just tank her up on IV fluids, give her antibiotics and get her in the OR. oseph and Mr. Wezzeh are here. Mr. Wezzeh doesn't seem too happy about the hospital closing.

"Someone shouldda ask us. If de hospital close, we lose de momentum we gain in de las' months. Wheh else des patients gonna go? We shoul' stay open."

Gillian comes to do the anesthesia and the spinal is quickly in. I scrub and Joseph preps the large abdomen. I make a slashing midline incision down to fascia and through into the subfascial tissues. I then tear them open to enter the peritoneal cavity. I quickly cut the rest of the fascia inferiorly and superiorly, lifting it up off the uterus with a finger while Mr. Wezzeh helps with his index.

I lift a bladder flap and push it down in the pelvis away from the uterus. Mr. Wezzeh protects it with a bladder retractor. I make a thin slice into the lower uterine segment and poke through with a clamp. I find placenta. I dig my fingers in until I can find a plane in the superior lateral aspect that is clear of placenta. Looks like she had a placenta previa as well.

I enlarge the uterine incision with scissors, grab the baby's two small feet and pull him out to his armpits. I then swing his anterior arm down and out, rotate him swiftly and extract his other arm, all the while keeping traction on the feet. I put a finger in his mouth pull the chin to his chest and deliver the fetal head.

The newborn is angry, too angry for words at first. I wipe him down quickly while Mr. Wezzeh clamps and cuts the cord. Almost as soon as I hand him off to Joseph he lets out a blood curdling yell!

I've never heard a newborn with lungs like these! His cries are piercing and a joy to my ears!

I close up and the woman goes back to her room. After washing the baby thoroughly, Gillian gives the baby the first dose of Nevirapine syrup to help prevent transmission of HIV from the mom. The mom will continue her anti-retrovirals.

I go downstairs and out to my apartment. I see some blood specks on my left scrub pant leg so I quickly strip down, dump my clothes in a tub of water, season it with antiseptic and take a bucket shower myself. Then I have some leftover rice, lentils and greens all mixed together in a delicious mash.

Next on the menu is Titus. He's our unofficial "PR man". After we saved his life, he got on national TV to say that the Cooper Hospital had done nothing for him. To emphasize his point he then lifted his shirt to reveal his colostomy with stool draining out into a colostomy bag. Very sensational for people who may have no idea that this is a temporary thing.

He's been prophylactically hospitalized since to keep him from embarrassing us and the government more in the media. He's actually turned into a nice, decent young man with the help of our chaplain.

As I come out of my office ready to go upstairs, Joseph from accounting accosts me.

"De Ministuh wanna see yo'."

"Sure, of course."

I go down the hallway towards the lobby where I'm met by a dignified, white haired man who introduces himself as the Minister of Health and a Surgeon.

"Ah'm concuhned 'bout de Coopuh Hospital closin'. You ha' been providin' a valuable suhvice to de community by stayin' open. We wanna know why you closin' and what will happen to de patients. De president especially ask me to find out 'bout Titus, de boy who wa' shot."

"Yeah, no problem. We're about to do his final procedure now. We are still taking care of our hospitalized patients until discharge. We're just not seeing or hospitalizing new patients."

"Yes, I hear fo' Titus it jus' a colostomy take down, raht? A simpuhl proseedhure…"

"That's right. He should be able to be discharged on Friday."

The Minister then ask about why we are closing. I tell him about R.B., the nurse's aide now in the Ebola unit at JFK. He starts to ask all kinds of questions. It seems to me he wants to convince us to only close for a few days and reopen as soon as possible.

I also realize I'm not the one he should be talking to. I refer him to Dr. Sonii, the medical director. They decide to wait for him, since he's already been called and is on his way. I go upstairs and prepare Titus for surgery with another IV line, IV fluids and antibiotics.

A short time later, we're ready to take down his colostomy. This time I give the spinal anesthetic and Gillian takes down the colostomy in a routine procedure. Nothing too exciting happens except I learn some cool suturing techniques for bowel and for colostomy skin wound closure.

I go check on Mr. Wennie who's been having TIA's and maybe a small stroke since yesterday. His blood pressure has been high. With no nurses on, I grab the BP cuff and go take Mr. Wennie's pressure myself.

It's low! 84/50! I grab some IV fluids and get a bolus going. He still is conscious if not quite his normal self. But then again, he hasn't been since yesterday. I also notice he has a slow heartbeat. I decide to stop his beta blocker. We'd put in a foley catheter earlier when we found out he had urinary retention. I confirm he has a huge prostate with a rectal exam. That may have been contributing to his resistant hypertension.

As you can see, the hospital is closed. But somehow I've still had a full day's work.

And I'm glad.

Rain

September 24

It's early in the morning. Rain is pouring down. The storm is pounding the corrugated roofs so loudly even thinking is difficult. Outside my office, the slums are abandoned. People have fled inside. The barbed wire twists along the top of the hospital compound's wall keeping it all on the outside. Now we are not only keeping intruders out, but patients as well.

I feel suddenly lost and without a purpose. I didn't come to Liberia for a vacation. I exposed myself to Ebola only because I felt I would be saving lives that otherwise might be lost. Now I wonder why I'm still here. Sure we have a c-section to do on Alex's wife who otherwise would be abandoned during our three weeks of closure. Of course, we have the post-op care on Titus after closing his colostomy. And we have a few other inpatients we have to tune up for discharge.

But mostly, since yesterday, I've been in a fog. My mind has suddenly become cloudy. I have no energy, no purpose. Even though I'm still here physically, mentally I've left. I was looking at pictures of my wife and kids yesterday and burst into uncontrollable sobbing. I'm ready to go home, but feel empty.

I didn't want to end my Liberia experience sitting around with too much time to analyze every little headache and wonder if I'm just a petri dish for Ebola at this point. It's one thing to take a risk for the benefit of others. It's another thing to just take a risk for no reason.

I wish the rain would just keep pouring down, somehow quarantining the Liberians and washing away Ebola forever. But according to some, it's already uncontainable. I certainly feel that's true if we stick to the current expensive methods. We'll just churn through the dollars and Ebola will just turn around and laugh, sticking it's tongue out at us laboring up the hill as he just disappears over the top.

It's so frustrating to leave, feeling like things are worse then when I came. Ebola is not slowing down, it's accelerating. The one hospital open to the public suffering from diseases other than Ebola is closed. And the Liberians are stuck. Me, I just get on a plane and leave it all behind (hopefully I'm not carrying Ebola with me). I can so easily move away and move on. But the West Africans can't escape the stress, the anxiety, the pressure, the fear, the plague, the pestilence, the economic disaster, the death all around.

Rain is so cleansing, why can't it just wash all this away...

Last Hurrah
September 27-28

The Cooper Hospital is closed, my clinical duties are finished. But I'm still in Liberia, what to do? It's Friday and I don't leave till Monday.

Paradise, here I come...again.

It's Saturday morning. Once again I find myself driving Gillian's Honda CRV out of Monrovia into the bush on the way to Robertsport. Once again, I'm accompanied by Robert and Abbie. This time, Gillian comes along bringing her tiny pseudo adopted son, Divine with us.

We stop in a roadside village and find potato greens boiled with plenty of chilis, palm oil and dried fish. We douse a big bowl of white rice with the greens and Robert, Abbie and I dig in with gusto. Gillian hates greens. My belly warmed, I finish driving the three hours to Robertsport.

I've brought some pictures of the young Liberians surfing from last week. I meet up with Morris who is thrilled. He takes me out to a left point break called Shipwrecks. I'm thankful for the 9'8" longboard that Dr. John from ELWA Hospital lent me as the waves are much smaller than last time.

Morris can't really catch anything with his shortboard, though he was tearing it up last week. He just has the perfect surfer vibe, though, a big smile on his face just being out in the water. I catch a steady stream of small, peeling, clean lefts and then call it a day.

Abbie and Robert want to make a bonfire. After downing some cold lentils and rice along with a peanut butter and jelly sandwich, I help them gather drift wood. We soon have a serious pile of all kinds and shapes of sticks. Robert and Abbie want to go watch Real Madrid play Chelsea at the video club in town. I take a nap. They come back two hours later after the sun has gone down accompanied by Morris. We soon have a roaring blaze going.

I start asking Morris a few simple questions. He starts talking easily, telling me the story of his life, how he got into surfing, and how he ended up being quarantined for Ebola.

When he was six years old, Morris was already helping his family fish. Sometimes they'd be out on the coast or on the islands for months at a time. His hands would become calloused from pulling the heavy ropes attached to the nets.

He'd see surfers out in the waves from time to time, though it was rare in those days. He started pretending to surf by taking a paddle from the fishing canoe and riding it down the sand cliffs formed as the tide wore away at a sand bank.

He'd been doing this awhile when a "whahte man" saw him one day and asked if he'd like to learn to surf. Morris, of course, agreed enthusiastically. The man gave him a basic lesson right there on the beach. Then he unleashed him with a board in the surf. On his first wave, Morris stood up, even though it was just for a few seconds.

He describes it as a miracle. He'd seen these guys flying across the water and it was miraculous. But then he found he was able to do it too. He was hooked. He started surfing almost every day. He was soon getting pretty good but felt that as a regular foot (left foot forward) he was handicapped. These exclusive left point breaks favor a goofy foot (right foot forward) approach. Morris decided to switch to goofy foot. His friends said he was crazy, but he was determined to take his surfing to the next level.

The first time he went out and tried to stand up goofy foot, he fell right off the board. Everyone laughed and mocked him. But Morris just smiled, paddled out to the line up and tried and tried again. That was in 2011. That same year, he won the Liberian surfing championship. He went on to take 2nd place in 2012 and 3rd place last year. This year, the competition was canceled due to the Ebola epidemic.

Grand Cape Mount County, with Robertsport as the county seat, had remained Ebola free until August. One woman then became sick, was quarantined and tested positive. They tried to quarantine her husband and daughter, but they fled into the bush. Both died, untested, but presumed positive. The woman was taken to Monrovia where she made a complete recovery. She lives just down main street.

Ebola panic began to set in. Everyone in the County who was sick or died was suspected to have had Ebola. St. Timothy's, the hospital on the hill originally built by the Episcopal Church and currently run by the government, closed down. There was no ambulance for the whole county. The lone doctor refused to work until the Ministry of Health sent him at least one ambulance so he could transfer patients to the capital if needed.

Then, Morris' oldest brother fell ill. He was a heavy smoker and 31 years of age. More seriously, according to Morris, he was stigmatized. In other words, someone cast a spell on him. He died shortly, thereafter. The County Public Health officials threw Morris and the rest of his family into quarantine for three weeks. The were locked in the local school and brought uncooked food, but nothing to cook it with. They were given no medicines and not even examined. Fortunately, after a week, they were released.

A few days later, another brother was stigmatized and died. Then a niece got a severe headache with fever one night. The next day she was dead. The family was placed back in quarantine under the same conditions, except this time they examined them and took some notes.

With no food or medicine, Morris was forced to use the $70 he'd been saving up for school—currently closed due to Ebola—to buy food and medicines for his family in quarantine. They were in quarantine for a total of six weeks. Morris just got out. When I surfed with him last week he'd just escaped the quarantine to come surf because he was going crazy being cooped up.

Of course, none of the family died or developed symptoms of any disease, much less Ebola. By now they had been quarantined for six weeks and had lost six weeks of fishing livelihood, not to mention Morris' life savings of $70.

By now, the fire is burning down. Morris gets up and goes to collect some more wood. Robert helps him and then we settle in for the night. Robert, Abbie and I share a thin blanket laid out under a tree. Gillian sleeps in the car with Divine. Morris stretches out right by the fire and keeps it stoked throughout the night.

In the middle of the night, it starts raining. Morris goes just up the beach to the big army tent he's sharing with a couple of guys. Robert, Abbie and I cram into the car. Abbie and I are in the front seats, Gillian and Divine in the back seat, and Robert in the rear hatchback storage area. Needless to say, it's a long, rough night with not much sleeping going on. It doesn't help that Divine is sick and cries most of the night.

With sunrise, Morris is back. He wants to show me a cave and some rock formations. We hike around the different capes and points, slog through thick sand, cross small streams, scramble over boulders and bushwhack through the jungle. I get shown two other "secret" breaks along the way. We find the rocks, but can't seem to find the cave. The trip has taken us one and a half hours. Then we hike the 90 minutes back. The surf still isn't great, but it looks promising at one of the "secret" spots called Locals.

Morris has to do something in town. While waiting for him to come back, I surf the beginner's break right in front of the car and catch a number of small, sweet little rides. Morris joins me on a beginner board and just goofs around, riding waves sitting down, standing on his head or lying down...all with a silly grin lighting up his face. We decide to go to Locals. I get out and walk. Morris paddles half way around before hitting the beach for the last stretch.

Locals isn't exactly pumping, but there are some good sized sets rolling in that give easy, relaxed yet big rides towards a boulder near the beach. Luckily, the wave seems to want to keep you away from the rocks. I enjoy some long rides until my arms are like jelly and incapable of paddling me out.

I say goodbye to Morris and we hit the road to Monrovia. I have only one more day in the Ebola Capital of the World.

Epilogue
September 29

Titus is recovering well. I removed his drain two days post op. He's eating, stooling and ambulating well. His wound is already shrinking. He was transferred this morning to a private room in the JFK Hospital. The President of Liberia wants him hospitalized until he's completely well. He still needs every other day dressing changes but otherwise has entirely recovered.

* * * * *

Mr. Wennie recovered his normal speech and neurologic function. It appeared his enlarged prostate was causing urinary retention leading to renal failure provoking uncontrollable hypertension making him almost have a stroke. I discharged him Wednesday, but he stayed in the hospital until today. He and Mrs. Wennie live in the same compound as Aaron. His body was finally taken away by the ministry of health on September 24. They did't test him for Ebola. His cadaver was either burned or dumped in a mass grave. We'll never know for sure, but always suspect he died of Ebola. The Wennies waited in the hospital until they'd finished spraying and disinfecting their compound.

* * * * *

Dr. Sonii came to my office and reported that his conscious is bothering him about the hospital closure. He especially feels for the OB patients. He's talked to some of the midwives who are willing to come back to work with some of the nurse's aides to help. He'll contract with a Congolese doctor who lives in the neighborhood to come do emergency c-sections until we can get a surgeon back full time. He hopes to reopen for obstetrics sometime next week.

* * * * *

Gillian is taking her long-overdue annual leave. She'll be back in early November.

* * * * *

I met with Dr. Moses from the Ministry of Health two days ago to talk about some economical, Liberian driven alternatives to the current NGO led losing battle against Ebola. He seemed receptive but pressured by the power wielded by the rich NGOs running the show. I fly back to California tonight rejoin my kids and pregnant wife.

* * * * *

R.B died Friday, September 26 in the JFK Hospital Ebola Treatment Unit. Her body was buried that afternoon.

* * * * *

Vivian was just admitted to the JFK ETU yesterday along with her husband. Both are positive for Ebola.

* * * * *

I have no idea what happened to Steve and his broken femur. He just disappeared.

* * * * *

Ebola Hemorrhagic Fever continues to run unchecked across West Africa and especially in Liberia. Some people estimate that it's already uncontainable and that there will be over a million cases by January 2015 if nothing is done differently to stem the tide...

The End (I wish)

Appendix
My Evil Plan to Eradicate Ebola from Liberia

I don't mean to be critical. I can't really know what's going on. I'm just a simple family doctor. I didn't really even take care of Ebola patients. How could I know why Liberia is losing the fight against Ebola? I haven't sat on any NGO committees or listened to the WHO discussions or what the CDC has to say. I'm just ignorant.

Right? But I'm going to give my opinion anyway.

Liberia is losing the fight against Ebola because they are depending on NGOs and an influx of Western money instead of traditional ways of dealing with epidemics. The first few Ebola epidemics were in remote villages. The villages touched by Ebola were self-quarantined according to ancient traditions of dealing with plagues.

No one went in and out and the surrounding communities brought them food. The caregivers washed themselves and their clothes quickly and frequently after each contact with the patient, just using simple soap and water. Many never got sick despite close contact with the virus. The epidemics were controlled within a few months.

In Liberia, everyone is excited about the millions of US dollars being poured in to "fight Ebola" and everyone wants a piece of the pie. A certain NGO out in rural Liberia quarantined a village, claiming they'd tested and found three cases. They applied for and received US$ 250,000 to fight Ebola in that village.

They brought in a few sacks of rice and some Chlorine. The villagers mobbed the trucks and carried off the plunder. And, miracle of miracles, not a single person died in the village. Great effort at treating and controlling Ebola? Or a scam in order to pocket some easy cash? I've never heard of a 0% fatality rate for Ebola, but you make the call.

MSF is spending hundreds of thousands of dollars to level earth with heavy equipment so they can build their Ebola Treatment Units. But it's taken them over a month to go from 120 beds to 140 beds when the 120 beds were saturated within days of opening. They are forced to turn hundreds away for lack of space. And the number of cases is multiplying exponentially.

Despite the millions of dollars being donated for the fight against Ebola, the patients aren't even being given IV fluids or adequate food. Which is why the Ebola patients sneak out of the tents and cross the street looking for something to eat. So much for isolation.

Dozens if not hundreds of $70,000 4x4 Land Cruisers with snorkels, large luggage wracks, heavy duty cattle grills, several spare tires, winches, and other off-road equipment are being used to take foreigners around the paved roads in town to hotels, bars, clubs, and fancy guest houses so they can feel comfortable while they fight Ebola

At the same time, they can't even collect the dead bodies that could expose so many more. We've had bodies left for up to 3 days. Others have stayed in the open for up to 5 days before being collected. The Red Cross comes screaming through Sinkor along 12th Street in front of the Cooper Hospital to pick up a single body using two brand new Hilux pickups, a Land Cruiser and a flat bed truck with about 10 people riding along. For a single body???

Patients are often turned away from the Ebola Treatment Units. MSF has even refused to take anyone who doesn't come in an ambulance. How many of the poor in West Point slum can afford an ambulance, even if there were enough available to take them?

I propose the following solution. I got the initial idea from an MSF doctor named Cameron. Improvements were suggested by Dr. John from ELWA.

There are three components to this simple, Liberian national-based solution to the Ebola question:

1. **Community-based Treatment Centers:**
    A. Infrastructure: each community, village or town, represented by its leaders should find a place that can be used to treat patients from their community. Schools are ideal because they are walled, have water and toilets and are currently empty because of the Ebola crisis.
    B. Staff: Individuals who have survived Ebola from the community should be recruited to care for the Ebola patients as they will be immune, not need special gear, and have no risk of furthering the spread of the virus. They should be paid at least

double a typical nurses salary and should sign a contract for three months renewable. They should be housed and fed on site so they can provide 24 hour care. Protective gear can be as simple as rain pants, rain jacket, rubber boots, long rubber gloves, and masks. The whole kit can be sprayed with chlorine between patients and reused.

C. Patients: suspect cases should be brought immediately to the treatment center and the Ministry of Health notified to send someone to draw their blood and test it for Ebola. The patient should not leave the treatment center or the community until he or she has been declared free of the virus by a negative test performed at least four days after the start of symptoms.

D. Medications & Supplies: the treatment centers should be provided with the following supplies:
1. ORS/water: enough for up to 6L per patient per day
2. Promethazine 25mg PO tid as needed for vomiting
3. Septrin 2 tabs PO bid x7 days
4. Artemether/Lumafantrine PO bid x 3 days
5. 3-4 bananas per patient per day (for K+ and Mg+)
6. Selenium 400mcg PO tid for the duration of symptoms
7. Chlorine in great quantity
8. Gloves, basins, towels, cleaning supplies, etc. etc. etc.

E. Quarantine: communities, led by their leaders, should quarantine those living in the same house as the Ebola suspected or confirmed patient. The community leaders should organize to provide food and water to those being quarantined for a period of at least two weeks.

2. **Testing for Ebola Hemorrhagic Fever**
A. Lab facilities: there should be enough lab supplies, lab techs and equipment to do at least 500 tests a day.
B. Phlebotomists: There should be at least 50 people able to draw blood safely off suspected patients. They should be ready to be deployed from 6AM to 6PM seven days a week. Community leaders will call the hotline to ask for a phlebotomist to come test a patient already held in the community treatment center or for dead bodies suspected of, but not diagnosed with Ebola.
C. Transport: the phlebotomists can go to the treatment centers via taxi to draw the blood and bring it back to the lab. Using taxis will stimulate the local economy and keep the money in working class Liberian hands instead of being invested in ex-pats' large Land Cruisers, drivers, hotel fees, restaurant/bar costs, salaries, plane tickets, etc.

3. **Collection and Disposal of Bodies**
   A. Transport: use local drivers with old beat-up pickups who would jump at the chance to make some money. Recruit at least 5 potential drivers in each community. There should be three to a team. Each one gets full protective gear. The team also gets a body bag and a chlorine water spray pump. Two team members put the body in the body bag after putting on all the protective gear. Then the third member sprays everything down including himself, the other team members and the body bag. Then the body is put in the truck and the protective gear taken off and disposed of appropriately
   B. Timely pick-up and delivery of bodies: the payment to the drivers for the bodies will be dependent on the rapidity of delivery of the body. I suggest the following sliding scale:

Time from call to Hotline to Delivery of Body	Wage Earned
Less than three hours	US $25
Three to six hours	US $20
Six to twelve hours	US $15
Twelve to twenty-four hours	US $10
Greater than twenty-four hours	US $5

   C. Crematoriums: There needs to be construction of more crematoriums until there is a capacity to handle at least 50 bodies a day. The corpses, once put in the body bags, are not reopened, examined or tested. Rather, they are put directly in the incinerator to be burned.

Conclusion:
With a much smaller amount of resources, with the participation of the communities and especially their leaders and with the distribution of resources among Liberian taxi drivers, Ebola survivors and truck drivers, the epidemic can be got under control by the Liberians themselves.

I'm not saying that there shouldn't be foreigners involved, I'm just saying the foreigners should be working alongside the Liberians helping them to find a solution to the Ebola problem. They shouldn't try to impose Western ideas that obviously aren't working. And it won't help in the long run to bring in a lot of money that will be spent on things that will just make the Liberians envious and want to share in the spoils of aid money.

About the Author

James Appel, MD holds a Bachelor of Arts in Theology from Southern Adventist University and a Doctor of Medicine from the Loma Linda University School of Medicine. He completed a three year residency in Family Practice at the Ventura County Medical Center in California. He has spent the last ten years working as a physician and surgeon in the Republic of Chad. James is married to a Danish nurse, Sarah, and together they have a daughter, Miriam, a son, Noah and another son, Isak, on the way.

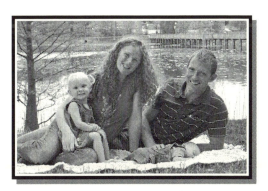

Made in the USA
Middletown, DE
05 February 2015